PUBLIC HEALTH IN THE 21ST CENTURY

DIARRHEA: OVERVIEW

PUBLIC HEALTH IN THE 21ST CENTURY

Additional books in this series can be found on Nova's website under the Series tab.

Additional E-books in this series can be found on Nova's website under the E-book tab.

PUBLIC HEALTH IN THE 21ST CENTURY

DIARRHEA: OVERVIEW

JOSHUA J. MALAGO

Nova Biomedical
Nova Science Publishers, Inc.
New York

Copyright © 2010 by Nova Science Publishers, Inc.

All rights reserved. No part of this book may be reproduced, stored in a retrieval system or transmitted in any form or by any means: electronic, electrostatic, magnetic, tape, mechanical photocopying, recording or otherwise without the written permission of the Publisher.

For permission to use material from this book please contact us:
Telephone 631-231-7269; Fax 631-231-8175
Web Site: http://www.novapublishers.com

NOTICE TO THE READER

The Publisher has taken reasonable care in the preparation of this book, but makes no expressed or implied warranty of any kind and assumes no responsibility for any errors or omissions. No liability is assumed for incidental or consequential damages in connection with or arising out of information contained in this book. The Publisher shall not be liable for any special, consequential, or exemplary damages resulting, in whole or in part, from the readers' use of, or reliance upon, this material.

Independent verification should be sought for any data, advice or recommendations contained in this book. In addition, no responsibility is assumed by the publisher for any injury and/or damage to persons or property arising from any methods, products, instructions, ideas or otherwise contained in this publication.

This publication is designed to provide accurate and authoritative information with regard to the subject matter covered herein. It is sold with the clear understanding that the Publisher is not engaged in rendering legal or any other professional services. If legal or any other expert assistance is required, the services of a competent person should be sought. FROM A DECLARATION OF PARTICIPANTS JOINTLY ADOPTED BY A COMMITTEE OF THE AMERICAN BAR ASSOCIATION AND A COMMITTEE OF PUBLISHERS.

Library of Congress Cataloging-in-Publication Data

Available upon request.
ISBN: 978-1-61728-830-2

Published by Nova Science Publishers, Inc. † New York

Contents

Preface		vii
Introduction		ix
Chapter I	Pathophysiology of the Different Types of Diarrhea	1
Chapter II	Etiological Agents of Diarrhea	9
Chapter III	Specific Causes of Diarrhea	15
Chapter IV	Special Forms of Diarrhea	41
Chapter V	Treatment of Diarrhea	45
Conclusion		51
References		53
Index		65

Preface

Diarrhea is a clinical symptom characterized by an increase in the volume, wateriness, or frequency of bowel movements. Diarrhea can be osmotic, secretory, malabsorptive, exudative, due to abnormal intestinal motility, or due to bacterial overgrowth.

In *osmotic* diarrhea, the gut mucosa fails to absorb intestinal contents into the blood stream resulting in accumulation of these substances in intestinal lumen. Subsequently, excessive amount of water remains in stool leading to diarrhea. Ingestion of non-absorbable materials, foods (e.g. some fruits and beans), sugars (e.g. hexitols, sorbitols) and accumulation of lactose in the intestine can cause osmotic diarrhea.

Secretory diarrhea develops following active secretion of electrolytes (sodium, chloride) and water by the intestines. It can be caused by toxins (e.g. cholera, *E. coli*), laxatives (e.g. castor oil), bile salts, fatty acids, and some tumors (e.g. carcinoid, gastrinoma).

Diarrhea due to *malabsorption* develops in people with malabsorption syndromes in which case normal digestion of food is impaired. The fat left in the intestinal lumen leads to secretory diarrhea while the carbohydrates cause osmotic diarrhea. It can also be due to nontropical sprue, pancreatic insufficiency, and inadequate blood supply to the large intestine.

Exudative diarrhea or inflammatory diarrhea follows destruction of the intestinal mucosa. The damaged intestinal mucosal cell leads to loss of fluid, proteins, mucous and blood as well as defective absorption of fluid and electrolytes. It is caused by infectious agents (e.g. *Shigella*), ulcerative colitis, Crohn's disease, tuberculosis, lymphoma, cancer, and viruses.

Diarrhea due to *abnormal motility* can be caused by hyperthyroidism, surgical removal of part of the intestine, cutting of vagus nerve, surgical bypass of part of the intestine, and drugs like antacids and laxatives containing magnesium, prostaglandins, serotonin, and caffeine.

Bacterial overgrowth as a cause of diarrhea is depicted when there is abnormal large numbers of normal intestinal bacteria (e.g. antibiotic associated pseudomembranous coli due to overgrowth of *Clostridium difficile*) or those normally not found in the intestines.

The causes of diarrhea can be infectious or non-infectious. Infectious causes are due to bacteria, viruses, or parasites and they can be noninflammatory when the enterocytes are not invaded or damaged, or inflammatory if enterocytic invasion and disruption by the pathogen has occurred. While watery diarrhea characterizes the noninflammatory type, blood, leucocytes, and pus are features of the stool in inflammatory diarrhea. Non-infectious diarrhea is watery in nature and results from various agents like heavy metal poisoning, laxatives and antacids containing metallic ions like Mg^{2+} and Na^+.

Treatment of diarrhea depends largely on the cause and duration. In acute cases, removal of the cause suppresses the diarrhea and the body heals by itself. When severe diarrhea causes dehydration, fluid therapy with water and electrolytes is done. Sometimes short term antidiarrheal drugs such as codein phosphate or loperamide are prescribed. The use of antibiotics can be advocated depending on the type of organism. In chronic cases, investigation (e.g. sigmoidoscopy, rectal biopsy) is needed prior to or with simultaneous symptomatic treatment.

Introduction

Diarrhea (Greek 'diarrhoia' = 'a flowing through') is a condition of having an increased frequency of loose or watery bowel movements. In a normal human population, bowel frequency ranges from three times a day to three times a week. Diarrhea is termed acute diarrhea when it lasts within 14 days; persistent diarrhea if it exceeds 14 days; and chronic diarrhea when the symptoms last longer than a month. While most cases of acute diarrhea are self limited, chronic cases need treatment.

Diarrhea is a worldwide problem. It constitutes a major cause of morbidity and mortality, especially among children, elderly, infirm, and immune compromised individuals. It is also more prevalent among adults who are exposed to children and non–toilet-trained infants, particularly in a daycare setting; in travelers to tropical regions; homosexual males; and people living in non-hygienic environments, with exposure to contaminated water or foods.

Both non-infectious and infectious agents can cause diarrhea although in the latter, the infecting organism(s) often cannot be identified. Invasive diarrhea occurs when the infecting pathogen crosses the intestinal mucosa. This may cause serious systemic symptoms. In some cases, invasive pathogens could even cause extra intestinal lesions. Viruses, particularly rotavirus and norovirus, are predominant diarrheal agents in developed countries while bacteria are the most frequent cause in developing region (Thapar and Sanderson 2004).

All the etiological agents of diarrhea converge at absorptive and secretory changes to increase the volume of water that enters the colon to a level beyond its absorptive capacity. This process, almost always arises as a result of one or more of the four basic mechanisms: osmotic diarrhea, secretory diarrhea, exudative diarrhea and diarrhea associated with motility disorders.

Chapter I

Pathophysiology of the Different Types of Diarrhea

Osmotic Diarrhea

Absorption of water in the intestine is dependent on adequate absorption of intestinal contents. When the gut fails to absorb intestinal contents into the blood stream, excessive amounts of solutes are retained in the intestinal lumen. The solutes raise the osmolarity and subsequently generate osmotic forces that retard the normal absorption of water or draws water into the lumen (Field 2003). Consequently, excessive amount of water remains in stool leading to osmotic diarrhea which is mainly watery in nature. Principally, osmotic diarrhea can result from the following two situations:

A. Ingestion of Non-Absorbable or Poorly Absorbed Substrates

In this case, the triggering molecule is usually a carbohydrate or a divalent ion. The carbohydrates can come from foods (e.g. some fruits and beans), sugars (hexitols, mannitol and sorbitols), and from accumulating lactose in the intestine (Oku et al 2008; Grabitske and Slavin 2009) (Table 1). These carbohydrates are osmotically active and can draw water into the intestinal lumen to cause diarrhea.

Table 1. Common foods that can cause diarrhea

Food	Ingredients causing diarrhea	Type of diarrhea
Apple and pear juices, sugar-free gums, mints	Hexitols, sorbitol, mannitol	Osmotic
Apple and pear juices, fruit flavors in soft drinks grapes, honey, dates, nuts,	Fructose	Osmotic
Table sugar	Sucrose	Osmotic
Milk, ice cream, yoghourt, soft cheese, chocolate	Lactose	Osmotic
Coffee, tea, and cola drinks	Caffein	Increased motility, secretory,

The second group of poorly absorbed substrates that are ingested are divalent ions from magnesium sulfate (Epsom salts), sodium sulfate, sodium phosphate, sodium citrate, and magnesium-containing antacids. These are the laxatives, antacids and saline purges prescribed for medications in several conditions (Fine et al 1991; Field 2003). The mechanisms of action of these ions centers at the repulsive behavior of similar charged molecules along the intestinal pores. Since the pores through which ions are absorbed are highly charged, the ions from these chemicals tend to be absorbed slowly. As a result, they accumulate within the intestinal lumen. Their accumulation raises the osmolality which in turn, slows and retards the normal absorption of water. Sometimes the osmolarity may be high enough to even draw water from the circulation into the intestinal lumen and thereby exacerbates further the diarrhea.

B. Maldigestion and Malabsorption

This refers to abnormal digestion and absorption of the ingesta in the intestine. Generally, any disease or condition that interferes with ingesta, especially osmotically active ingesta like carbohydrate, will lead to osmotic diarrhea. It can be due to losses of digestive enzymes that lead to maldigestion and subsequent malabsorption of nutrients (Layer et al 1997). This disorder is exemplified by lactase deficiency that is manifested as lactose intolerance, a condition often developing after weaning in many individuals (He et al 2008). In such cases, consumed lactose (usually as milk) cannot be effectively hydrolyzed into glucose and galactose for absorption. The unabsorbed lactose accumulates in the intestinal lumen, becomes osmotically active and retains water in the small intestine leading to osmotic diarrhea. The same mechanism applies for impaired intraluminal digestion due to pancreatic insufficiency and small bowel disease that cause secondary disaccharidase deficiencies (Pezzilli 2009).

The unabsorbed carbohydrates are anaerobically fermented in the colon by the intestinal microbioata leading to production of intermediary products (ethanol and formic, succinic and lactic acids) as well as short-chain fatty acids (SCFA) (acetate, propionate, and butyrate) (Malago et al 2003). The intermediary products are converted to produce CO_2 and H_2 that are rapidly absorbed. Excessive production of gas causes borborygmus and flatus rich in H_2. The SCFA can be absorbed from the colon to serve as source of energy to the colonocytes. However, these acids are osmotically active and can contribute to diarrhea when their concentration in the colon is high as it is in severe carbohydrate malabsorption (He et al 2008).

Treatment

Abstaining from ingesting poorly or no-absorbable carbohydrates or solutes stops the clinical symptoms of osmotic diarrhea.

Secretory Diarrhea

Under normal conditions, the small intestine secretes as well as absorbs fluid and electrolytes. The secretion rate is lower than the absorption rate and thus the net effect is absorption of fluid. Pathophysiologic events that reduce the absorption rate by either stimulating secretion or inhibiting absorption lead to secretory diarrhea, which is mainly watery. The most common cause of this type of diarrhea is a cholera toxin that stimulates the secretion of anions, especially chloride ions. Then, to maintain a charge balance and osmolarity in the lumen, sodium is carried with the chloride, along with water. The net result is increased water and electrolyte in intestinal lumen and the subsequent watery diarrhea (Field 2003; Alam and Ashraf 2003; Sack et al 2004). Principally, all the fluid secreted into or absorbed from the lumen of the small intestine during the digestive process flows across the mucosa in response to osmotic gradients. Since perturbations of absorption and secretion lead to secretory diarrhea, it is important to get an overview on the events of these processes before discussing the development of the diarrhea.

Intestinal Absorption

As a rule of thumb, absorption of ingesta in the small intestine is a tight coupling between water and solute, particularly Na^+. There are several mechanisms by which Na^+ is absorbed into the cell but the most common is by cotransport with glucose and amino acids. As the absorbed Na^+ accumulates in the cell, large amount of it is pumped out of the cell via sodium pump into the intercellular spaces between adjacent enterocytes where it establishes a high osmolarity. Subsequently, water diffuses into the intercellular space in response to the osmotic gradient established by Na^+. Some of the water diffuses through the tight junctions (Fordtran et al. 1968; Binder 1977; Edmonds 1984; Russo et al 2003). Absorption is completed by diffusion of both water and Na^+ into capillary blood within the villus.

Intestinal Secretion

Two distinct processes have been established to be involved in the secretion of water into the lumen of the intestine.

A. Increases in Luminal Osmotic Pressure by Digested Foodstuffs

Digestion of the macromolecules of the chyme that floods into the intestine from the stomach produces thousands of osmotically active molecules (e.g. maltose, glucose, amino acids). These molecules increase osmolarity of intestinal lumen. The increased luminal osmolarity stimulates secretion of water by pulling it into the lumen. Then, as the osmotically active molecules are absorbed, osmolarity of the intestinal contents decreases and water, together with nutrients, can be absorbed (Fordtran et al 1968; Binder 1977; Edmonds 1984).

B. Active Secretion of Electrolytes by Crypt Cells

The apical membrane of crypt epithelial cells contains cyclic adenosine monophosphate (cAMP)-dependent Cl^- channel responsible for secretion of water. The secretion process starts by Cl^- entry into the crypt epithelial cell by cotransport with Na^+ and K^+. Na^+ is pumped back out via Na^+ pumps while K^+ is exported via a number of channels. This is followed by activation of adenyl cyclase leading to generation and accumulation of cAMP in crypt cells that in turn, activates the cAMP-dependent chloride channel resulting in secretion of Cl^- into the lumen. In addition, accumulation of Cl^- in the crypt creates an electric potential that attracts Na^+, pulling it into the lumen across tight junctions. The net result is secretion of NaCl into the crypt and the lumen. NaCl secretion in the crypts creates an osmotic gradient across the tight junction and water is drawn into the lumen (Fordtran et al 1968; Binder 1977; Edmonds 1984; Russo et al 2003).

Perturbations of absorption and secretion known to cause secretory diarrhea may involve bacterial toxins (both heat-labile and heat-stable toxins), hormones and peptides acting locally (e.g. paracrine hormones), neurotransmitters, prostaglandins, materials in intestinal lumen (e.g. bile acids and fatty acids), and intestinal physical factors (e.g. intestinal distention due to obstruction or ileus. This produces secretion proximal to the obstruction as tight junctions are stretched and broken leading to increased permeability). Other factors and their produced active substances in brackets include Zollinger-Ellison syndrome (gastrin), pancreatic cholera syndrome (vasoactive intestinal peptides), medullary carcinoma of the thyroid (calcitonin), glucagonomas (glucagon), and malignant carcinoid syndrome (serotonin) (Metz 1999; Field 2003; Navaneethan and Giannella 2008; Pezzilli 2009; Tormo et al 2009; Zimmer et al 2009). Although the exact diarrheal mechanisms for these factors remain enigmatic, they revolve around stimulating crypt secretion (e.g. prostaglandins), increasing intestinal permeability, and altering intestinal functional morphology. In some cases, the active agents do not impair the colonocytic absorption activity. Rather, the colon may be unable to adequately reabsorb the fluid load when the secretion in the small bowel is so massive.

Patients with secretory diarrhea will have large-volume watery stool (above 1 L/day) without excessive fat, blood or pus. And because of water and electrolyte secretion, the patients will be depleted of fluid, and electrolyte (mainly Na^+ and K^+).

Generally, secretory diarrhea can be treated by removing the offending agent and oral fluid (particularly glucose-saline) replacement for maintenance of hydration. Cholestyramine is indicated for bile acid-induced diarrhea.

Secretory diarrhoeas, mostly acute and due to infections (bacteria, viruses, parasites), are by far the most important subtype of diarrheas in terms of frequency, incidence and mortality (over 2.5 million deaths/year) (Baldi et al 2009).

Exudative or Inflammatory Diarrhea

This type of diarrhea follows structural destruction of the intestinal mucosal lining or brush border by diffuse ulceration, inflammation, infiltrations, and tumors. The damaged intestinal mucosal cell leads to loss of fluid, serum proteins, mucous and blood as well as defective absorption of fluid and electrolytes (Field 2003). There is also addition of pus (cellular debris, inflammatory cells and pathogenic bacteria) to the intestinal lumen. The effects on stool volume and composition are most pronounced when the lesions also involve the colon, since there will be little opportunity for normal mechanisms of colonic fluid and electrolyte absorption to compensate for the increased volume of chime (Field 2003; Navaneethan and Giannella 2008; Baldi et al 2009). This type of diarrhea is observed in shigellosis, ulcerative colitis, Crohn's disease, tuberculosis, lymphoma, enteric (especially colon) cancers, and viral and parasitic infections.

Diarrhea due to Abnormal Motility

Diarrhea due to abnormal intestinal motility is caused by rapid movement of food through the intestines (hypermotility). The intestinal hypermotility reduces the absorption time for nutrients and water leading to diarrhea. It can be caused by hyperthyroidism, surgical removal or surgical bypass of part of the intestine, cutting of vagus nerve, complications of menstruation, and drugs like antacids and laxatives containing magnesium, prostaglandins, serotonin, and caffeine (Field 2003; Navaneethan and Giannella 2008; Baldi et al 2009). This type of diarrhea can be treated with antimotility agents such as loperamide.

The Pathophysiology

Motility of the small intestine is controlled by contractile intestinal motor activity interposed with periods of quiescence. This activity governs the rate at which materials travel along the intestine to the anus as well as the time and thus the degree of contact between the ingesta, the digestive enzymes, and the absorptive epithelium. Hormones, such as motilin, neurotensin, cholecystokinin and vasoactive intestinal peptide (VIP) are also involved in inducing intestinal hypermotility particularly in acute infectious gastroenteritis (Tormo et al 2008). The increase in intestinal motility limits digestion and absorption of gut contents by accelerating transit of materials leading to diarrhea (Layer et al 1997). Premature evacuation of the colon and surgical removal of ileocecal sphincter are good examples of this type of diarrhea. To understand the latter example, a brief overview of the functional morphology of the ileocaecal sphincter is needed. In human, the ileocecal sphincter is about 4 cm long at the distal small intestine. It produces high-pressure zone (about 20 mm Hg) that plays role in regulating intestinal transit. When the ileum distends, the ileocecal sphincter pressure decreases to allow intestinal transit across the sphincter, whereas distention of the colon increases the sphincter pressure to slow down intestinal transit and prevent backwash from the colon. Surgical removal of the ileocecal sphincter leads to increased intestinal transit and potential for bacterial overgrowth from fecal backwash (Quigley and Phillips 1983; Nasmyth and Williams 1985; Johnston et al 1989). Both increased intestinal transit and bacterial overgrowth result in diarrhea.

Chapter II

Etiological Agents of Diarrhea

The etiological agents of diarrhea can be divided into infectious and non-infectious. Infectious agents are mainly bacteria of various species and strains, viruses, and parasite.

Bacterial Diarrhea

Most acute bacterial diarrheas are self-limiting and usually resolve within two weeks. They can, depending on the pathogenetic mechanisms, be classified into toxigenic and invasive types. In toxigenic bacterial diarrheas an enterotoxin is the major pathogenic mechanism while in invasive types the organism invades the enterocyte with or without subsequent production of an enterotoxin. Bacterial enterotoxins can either produce intestinal fluid secretion by activating intracellular enzymes without damage to the epithelial surface, e.g. *Vibrio cholerae*, some strains of *E. coli*, and *Bacillus cereus* (cytotonic) or can injure the enterocytes and induce fluid secretion, e.g. *Shigella* and *Salmonella* (cytotoxic) (Table 2).

Acute bacterial etiology occurs in 1.5%-5.6% of acute diarrhea cases in adult humans. The most frequently identified organisms are *Campylobacter* (2.3%), *Salmonella* (1.8%), *Shigella* (1.1%) or *Escherichia Coli* (0.4%). When an invasive bacterium is present (e.g. *Shigella spp*, *Salmonella spp*) fever and bloody diarrhea are often observed. The pathogens are normally ingested, overtake the immune system, and adhere to the intestinal wall. They then invade the cells and or produce toxins that alter the metabolism of the cell. The invaded cells die and both the bacteria and toxins can invade bloody circulation to cause systemic symptoms like fever, chills, hypotension, nausea and vomiting (Navaneethan and Giannella 2008; Baldi et al 2009). Figure 1 depicts some of the ways by which bacteria cause diarrhea.

Table 2. Bacterial causes of diarrhea and their pathogenic mechanisms

Pathogenic mechanisms	Non-inflammatory	Inflammatory
I. Preformed enterotoxin	Staphylococcus aureus, Bacillus cereus	-
II. Enterotoxigenic,	ETEC, Vibrio cholera, Vibrio parahaemolyticus, Clostridium perfringens	Shigella, EIEC, Yersinia, Campylobacter, Salmonella, Clostridium difficile
III. Enteroadherent		
A. Attaching and effacing		EPEC, EHEC
B. Noneffacing		EAEC, DAEC, S. Typhimurium
IV. Invasive		
A. Superficial mucosal invasion		Shigella spp., EIEC
B. Submucosal invasion		Yersinia enterocolitica, Campylobacter jejuni Salmonella serovars; e.g., Typhi and Paratyphi

Viral Diarrhea

Viruses such as Norovirus (formerly Norwalk virus) and rotavirus grow in the small intestine and destroy absorptive villous epithelial cells but not crypt epithelium or lamina propria. The destruction causes villous atrophy. Both digestive and absorptive capacities of the mucosa are reduced because of diminished villous surface area, numbers of absorptive cells, and functional capacity of the remaining incompletely differentiated cells (Anderson and Weber 2004; Tormo et al 2008). The ingesta and alimentary secretions are not digested or absorbed but rather undergo bacterial degradation and fermentation. This degradation increases the osmolarity of the intestinal contents, and fluid is drawn into the intestine by the resultant osmotic gradient (Tormo et al 2008). Often the viruses do not affect absorptive cells in the large intestine. However, the damage in the small intestine causes the materials presented to the large intestine to be qualitatively abnormal and its quantity exceeds the absorptive capacity of the large intestine.

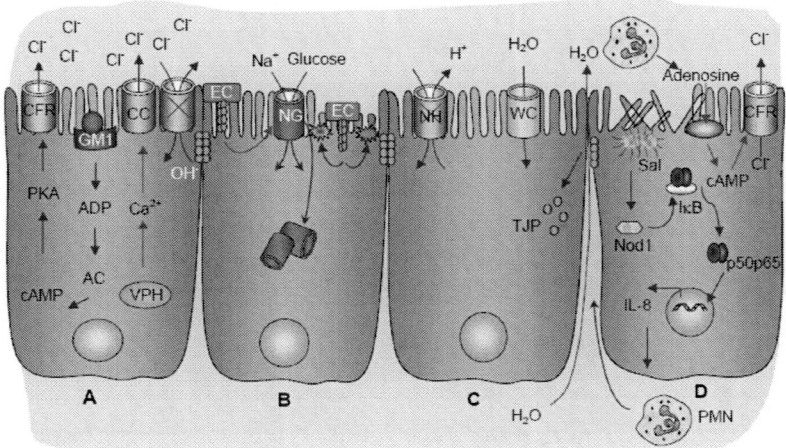

Figure 1.
A. Vibrio bacteria induce secretion of Cl⁻ by small intestinal epithelial cells. The cholera toxin secreted by *Vibrio cholera* is bound to the GM1 receptor on the cell membrane. This is followed by induction of ADP-ribosylation of adenylate cyclase which subsequently activates cAMP. In turn cAMP activates protein kinase A (PKA), which phosphorylates the cystic fibrosis transmembrane receptor (CFR) leading to Cl⁻ secretion. Secreted *V. parahemolyticus* thermostable direct haemolysin (VPH) activates Ca^{2+} which leads to Cl⁻ secretion by the calcium-activated chloride channels (CC). Inhibition of Cl⁻ absorption also occurs in both organisms.
B. Enteropathogenic *Escherichia coli* (EC) decreases apical Na^+, Cl⁻, and glucose absorption through two ways; first by causing movement of apical Na^+/glucose cotransporter (NG) into intracellular vesicles and second by effacing (wiping) microvilli and hence loss of NG. Both mechanisms depend on injection of effector proteins.
C. Na^+ absorption can be decreased following inhibition of the Na+/H+ exchanger 3 (NH). Further, direct inhibition of water channels (WC) can occur in the course of diarrhea. Water can also accumulate in the lumen following disruption of tight junctions.
D. Invasive organisms like Salmonella (Sal) cause membrane ruffling, stimulate Nod1 pathway that activate inhibitory kappa B to release p50-p65 molecules that translocate intranuclearly to activate proinflammatory cytokine production, especially interleukin (IL)-8. Secreted IL-8 attracts polymorphonuclear cells (PMN) that release 5'-AMP that is converted to adenosine which activates cAMP in the cell to activate the CFR leading to Cl⁻ secretion.

Parasitic Diarrhea

Intestinal parasitic infections account for 20%-25% of infectious diarrhoeas, which are mostly chronic and endemic in developing countries (Ball et al. 1996). They can be divided into three groups; protozoa, roundworms and flatworms. The flatworms may be further divided into cestodes (tapeworms) and trematodes (flukes). Only few significant parasites will be discussed here.

The protozoans *Giardia lamblia, Cryptosporidium parvum,and Entamoeba histolytic* form the most important diarrhea causing parasites in humans. *Blastocystis hominis* and *Ascaris lumbricoides* are less popular parasites but quite often associated with diarrhea in children (Carvalho-Costa et al. 2007; Tormo et al. 2008).

Other parasitic conditions that can cause diarrhea during parasitic life in the human host include Ascaris, Trichuris,Strongyloides, Filariasis, Toxocara, Echinococcosis, Cysticercosis, Tapeworms, Trematoda, Schistosoma, and hook worm. The symptoms may considerably vary among the species and becoming more severe in children (Carvalho-Costa et al. 2007; Tormo et al. 2008). In general terms, they will be characterized by chronic diarrhea and abdominal pains. Antihelmintics will treat the illnesses.

Non-Infectious Causes

Non-infectious causes of diarrhea are caused by several unrelated agents and conditions. They normally result in watery diarrhea and vomiting. Good examples include acute heavy metal poisoning due to ingestion of copper, zinc, iron or cadmium. These agents may cause nausea, vomiting, cramps and diarrhea occurring 5 to 60 minutes after ingestion (Bishai et al. 1993). Probably the largest group of non-infectious diarrhea is the diarrhea due drug use. There are more than 700 drugs that have been implicated in causing diarrhea through various mechanisms. They include altered gastrointestinal defenses, mucosal damage of the small and large intestine and/or disruption of normal processes of fluid and electrolyte absorption and secretion; sometimes more than one mechanism may be involved (Ratnaike and Jones 1998). Drugs containing Mg^{+2} e.g antiacids and laxatives; antiarrhythmic drugs such as quinidine, procainamide and disopyramide; colchicines administered for acute gout; and antimetabolites like methotrexate cause diarrhea as a side effect, in different ways. In elderly individuals, the most common drugs associated with diarrhea include antibiotics, proton pump inhibitors, allopurinol, psycholeptics, selective serotonin reuptake inhibitors and the antihypertensive angiotensin II receptor blockers.

In most cases the non-infectious diarrhea will resolve with discontinuance of the drug or chemical.

Chapter III

Specific Causes of Diarrhea

Infectious Diarrhea

Non-Inflammatory Diarrhea

The aetiological agents of non-inflammatory diarrheas do not cause considerable acute intestinal inflammation or mucosal destruction. Instead they alter the absorptive and/or secretory processes of the enterocyte after adhering to small intestinal mucosa. As a result, they cause large-volume watery diarrhea without blood, leukocytes, pus, or tenesmus. Nausea, vomiting, and abdominal pains can be experienced but without fever. Examples of these agents are *Vibrio cholera, Vibrio parahaemolyticus, Enterotoxigenic E. coli (ETEC), Clostridium perfringens, Bacillus cereus, Staphylococcus aureus,* Norovirus, Rotavirus, *Giardia lamblia,* and *Cryptosporidia parvum.*

Bacteria

Vibrio Cholerae

Vibrio cholerae is the prototypic cause of toxigenic diarrhea. Every year more than 100,000 cholera cases and 2000-3000 deaths are officially reported to WHO (Baldi et al 2009). The organism's natural habitat is estuarine and coastal waters, where it can be found living free and associated with invertebrates. Infection occurs following ingestion of food or water contaminated with the bacteria.

Following ingestion, *V. cholera* must adhere to the proximal small intestinal (e.g. the duodenum and upper jejunum) mucosa to survive. The adherence is mediated by a fimbrial colonization factor, known as the toxin-coregulated pilus (Sack et al. 2004). There could be other pilus structures like the fucosebinding and mannose-binding hemagglutinins that may also promote colonization by different *V. cholerae* biotypes (Shogomori and Futerman 2001). After adhesion, *V. cholera* secretes the cholera toxin which is the principal virulence factor.

The secreted cholera toxin consists of two subunits, a single toxic active A subunit (CTA), and a binding B subunit (CTB), which binds the toxin to the enterocytes via a brush border membrane ganglioside (GM1) receptor (Shogomori and Futerman 2001). The bound toxin is internalized into the enterocytes where the A subunit is cleaved into A1 and A2 peptides. The A1 peptide has enzymatic ADP-ribosylating activity and thus stimulates the ribosylation of Gs leading to activation of adenylate cyclase (Sack et al. 2004). Activated adenylate cyclase then elevates cAMP which subsequently stimulates the intestinal crypt cells to secrete chloride and fluid while at the same time blocking sodium, chloride, and fluid absorption in the villous cells. The end result is voluminous fluid efflux into the intestinal lumen and the subsequent severe acute watery diarrhea (Sack et al 2004). Additionally, the cholera toxin stimulates enterochromaffin cells to release serotonin, which in turn stimulates the release of vasointestinal peptide from local enteric neurons, also producing diarrhea (Mourad et al. 1995).

The *V. cholerae* diarrhea stool, 'rice water', output can exceed 1 L/hour. This massive outpouring of electrolyte-rich isotonic fluid into the bowel and out of the body often leads to volume depletion and shock, followed by renal and cardiac failure.

Treatment is based on restoring fluid and electrolyte balance either intravenous or oral, and maintaining intravascular volume. This therapy decreases the number of deaths from 50% to less than 1% (Marcos and DuPont, 2007). Even though fluid and electrolyte transport is impaired, glucose transport is intact. Since glucose absorption carries Na^+ and subsequently Na^+ goes with water, an oral rehydration solution containing glucose, sodium and water will enhance water absorption in dehydration stage of cholera.

Vibrio Parahaemolyticus

Vibrio parahaemolyticus is a halophilic (salt-requiring) bacterium naturally and commonly found in warm marine and estuarine environments. It commonly infects oysters and seafood. The bacterium causes acute diarrheal disease after consumption of seafood especially raw or undercooked fish or shellfish, particularly oysters. The common factor in most outbreaks appears to be storage of the food for several hours without proper refrigeration (Cabello et al. 2007). Less commonly, *V. parahaemolyticus* can cause an infection in the skin when an open wound is exposed to warm seawater. Watery diarrhea is the cardinal manifestation along with gastrointestinal symptoms, abdominal cramping, nausea, vomiting, fever, and chills. Most persons recover after 3 days and suffer no long-term consequences. The disease can be fatal in people with cirrhosis (Hally et al 1995). Treatment is symptomatic and there is no role for antimicrobial therapy.

Enterotoxigenic E. Coli (ETEC)

Enterotoxigenic *E. coli*, ETEC, colonizes the proximal small intestine after passing through the acid barrier of the stomach. They colonize the surface without penetrating the mucus layer. Like cholera, ETEC do not cause significant histological damage to the epithelium nor bacteremia. Further, it causes a less severe diarrhea than *V. cholerae*. Detailed studies have indicated that ETEC are positioned 50-100 nm from the microvilli of plasma membrane. They are thought to colonize the epithelial cell glycocalyx, a carbohydrate rich coat under the mucous layer that covers the surface of the epithelium, rather than the plasma membrane itself. Adherence and attachment to the mucosal is through ligand-receptor interaction via protein antigens on the surface of fimbriae (Evans et al. 1975). This colonization is followed by elaboration of heat-labile or heat-stable toxin or both to cause clinical disease. The heat-stable toxin stimulates intestinal crypt cell secretion of chloride and fluid and blockade of intestinal villous absorption of sodium and fluid through guanylate cyclase and subsequently cGMP. About half of clinical isolates of ETEC secrete heat-stable enterotoxin only (Wolf 1997).

The heat-labile toxin produces diarrhea by activating adenylate cyclase through ADP ribosylation of Gs (Moss and Richardson 1978) that elevates intracytoplasmic cAMP as does *V. cholerae*.

The disease begins after 24 to 48 hours of ingestion of contaminated food or water with upper abdominal distress followed by watery diarrhea. The infection can be mild (with only a few loose movements) or severe as in cholera.

Treatment for E. Coli

In most of the *E. coli* infections (not only of ETEC), treatment is symptomatic and involves correction of fluid and electrolytes in dehydrating individuals. Antibiotic therapy is ineffective and favors the emergence of resistant strains. However, in severe cases of enterohaemorrhagic *E. coli* (EHEC) with possible toxic megacolon, systemic antibiotics are advocated. For cramping and diarrhea, bismuth subsalicylate may be given. For infants and immunocompromised patients, intravenous antibiotics based on the organism's drug sensitivity and salicylates or opium tincture for cramping and diarrhea can be given. Antidiarrheals, such as loperamide, should be avoided in *E. coli* infections.

Clostridium Perfringens

Clostridium perfringens is a spore-forming bacterium and a natural inhabitant of soil and the intestinal tract of many warm-blooded animals and humans. The organisms causes diarrhea in two different food borne diseases namely Type A diarrhea and Type C human necrotic enteritis (Granum 1990).

Type A diarrhea is relatively mild and more common in the industrialized world. Infection follows ingestion of at least 10^7 *C. perfringens* spores from contaminated heat-treated food. The heat-treated food kills competing intestinal microbioata while the *C. perfringens* spores survive, vegetate and multiply to dominate the gut flora. The bacterium then produces the enterotoxin (CPE) type A that causes the illness (Skelkvåle and Uemura 1977; Sarker et al 1999). A similar mechanism occurs following uptake of antibiotics that kill off most members of the gut microbiota to pave way to multiplication of *C. perfringens*. Thus the pathogen is also an important cause of antibiotic associated diarrhea through induction of type A toxin (Sparks et al 2001).

The symptoms develop about 6–24 hours after eating contaminated food and they last 12-24 hours. They include acute abdominal pain, nausea and watery diarrhea. A severe life-threatening necrotizing enterocolitis can also develop (Rood and Cole 1991; Dittmar et al 2008).

C. perfringens type C food poisoning is a very serious but rare disease (Granum 1990). In this disease, the ingested spores from contaminated food develop into vegetative form that produce b-toxin (major disease agent) as well as d- and q-toxins (Jolivet-Reynaud et al 1986; Granum 1990). The disease is associated with individuals having low levels of proteolytic enzymes in their intestines often caused by low protein intake. Further, the disease can develop after eating diets containing trypsin inhibitors which prevent degradation of b-toxin. Normally the toxin is inactivated by the normal trypsin activity in the duodenum and small intestine (Steinthorsdottir et al. 2000).

Symptoms of *C. perfringens* type C food poisoning develop after 5–6 hours of ingestion of the spores. They start with an acute sudden onset of severe abdominal pain and bloody diarrhea, with or without vomiting, followed by necrotic inflammation of the small intestine. The disease is fatal if not treated and if treated, the mortality rate falls to 15–25%.

Antimicrobial therapy is generally not recommended. C. perfringens foodborne diseases can be controlled via proper cleaning and disinfection although large outbreaks, sometimes with fatal outcomes are still frequently reported (Labbé 2000).

Bacillus Cereus

Bacillus cereus is a spore-forming organism ubiquitous in nature and is part of the intestinal flora of different animals. Like *C. perfringens*, it is a common cause of food borne disease by virtue of its highly adhesive endospores, spreading to all kinds of foods. The bacterium causes two types of gastrointestinal disease, the diarrhoeal and the emetic syndromes, which are caused by different types of toxins.

The emetic syndrome is caused by a small ring-formed peptide, cereulide, preformed during vegetative growth of the bacterium in contaminated food (Ehling-Schulz et al. 2004). After ingestion and release from the stomach into the duodenum, it is suggestive that the toxin binds to the $5-HT_3$ receptor, and stimulates the vagus afferent causing vomiting (Agata et al. 1995). Emetic syndrome develops following ingestion of starch-rich foods such as fried and cooked rice, pasta, pastry and noodles. Symptoms occur about 0.5-6 hours and are characterized by nausea, vomiting and malaise. A few lethal cases, possibly due to liver damage, also occur (Ehling-Schulz et al 2004; Arnesen et al. 2008).

The diarrhoeal type of food poisoning is caused by a single protein, a cytotoxin (CytK) (Lund et al 2000), and two other enterotoxin complexes; one of these, a nonhaemolytic enterotoxin (Nhe), consists of three components (NheA, NheB, and NheC) (Lund and Granum 1996) and the second complex, haemolysin BL (HBL) (Beecher et al. 1995) contains the protein components B, L_1 and L_2. The diarrhea toxins are produced during vegetative growth of *B. cereus* in the small intestine (Granum 1994). They cause rapid disruption of the plasma membrane and formation of pores in planar lipid bilayers to cause diarrhea (Fagerlund et al. 2008).

The diarrhea syndrome follows ingestion of proteinaceous foods like meat products, soups, vegetables, puddings, sauces, milk and milk products. Symptoms occur about 8-16 hours and last approximately 24 hours. They include abdominal pain, profuse watery diarrhea and occasionally nausea. Lethality has occurred (Arnesen et al. 2008)

Both types of food poisoning develop following ingestion of food that has been heat-treated and cooled. *B. cereus* spores survive and grow well after cooking and cooling to tepmperatures below 48°C and thus serve as good source of the food poisoning. Contrary to *C. perfringens*, *B. cereus* is not a competitive micro-organism.

The *B. cereus* infections are self limiting and antimicrobial therapy is not recommended.

Staphylococcus Aureus

Staphylococcus aureus diarrhea manifests in two ways; food borne and antibiotic associated diarrhea. In both cases, *S. aureus* enterotoxins are the principal agents involved.

Staphylococcal food poisoning is characterized by sudden onset of abdominal cramps, nausea, vomiting, and diarrhea and in a minority of cases, fever. About 50% of the victims may need hospitalization. Symptoms develop shortly after ingestion of preformed toxin which is usually in foods that are cooked (e.g. ham or omelet) and then improperly stored at room temperature (Holmberg and Blake 1984). Outbreaks can also follow contamination of food by food handlers with *S. aureus* infected lesions.

In antibiotic associated diarrhea, the enterotoxigenic *S. aureus* occasionally found in the human gastrointestinal tract without any bowel symptoms (Lindberg et al. 2000; Ray et al. 2003), induces a sporadic and nosocomial diarrhea following antibiotic therapy (Naik et al. 2008; Lis et al. 2009). The antibiotic therapy alters the gut microbioata leading to expression of pathogenic properties of the intestinal *S. aureus* (Donskey 2004). Many of these pathogens produce toxins such as enterotoxins A, C, or D, leucotoxins LukE, LukD, or toxic shock syndrome toxin 1 (Gravet 1999; Asha et al. 2006; Flemming and Ackermann 2007) responsible for the illness. Continual use of the antibiotics leads to emergency of antibiotic resistant *S. aureus* strains such as the methicillin-resistant *S. aureus*. The antibiotic-resistant pathogen spreads and multiplies to reach even 10^8 $CFUg^{-1}$ when most of the competing microbioata are eliminated under antibiotic pressure. Clinically, the antibiotic resistant strains cause a more severe illness in terms of duration of diarrhea, number of bowel movements, and total volume of stool, than non resistant *S. aureus* strains (Boyce and Havill 2005).

Because the symptoms of *S. aureus* associated diarrhea are due to preformed toxins and are self-limited, antimicrobial therapy is not recommended.

Viruses

Norovirus

Norovirus causes approximately 90% of epidemic non-bacterial outbreaks of gastroenteritis around the world. It affects people of all ages (Ciarlet and Estes 2001). The viruses are transmitted by faecally contaminated food or water and by person-to-person contact. Airborne transmission due to aerosolisation of the viruses from vomiting patients stricken with the virus individuals has also been reported. Further, infection can follow eating food near an episode of vomiting, even if cleaned up. Norovirus is highly contagious, with as few as ten virus particles being able to cause infection. Outbreaks often occur in closed or semi-closed communities, such as long-term care facilities, overnight camps, hospitals, prisons, dormitories, and cruise ships.

Norovirus causes broadening and blunting of intestinal villi and exerts a direct action on the activity of enzymes of the brush border by diminishing the activity of intestinal disaccharidases (Musher and Musher 2004). These events lead to malabsorption and diarrhea.

The Norovirus causes a self-limiting syndrome with an incubation period of 1 to 2 days. It is associated with a variable combination of fever, anorexia, nausea, vomiting, myalgia, abdominal pain and diarrhea. The vomiting represents delayed gastric emptying; there are no morphologic features of gastritis. Spontaneous recovery occurs two to three days later. Severe illness is rare but the disease is fatal in very young, elderly, and persons with weakened immune systems (Nakagomi et al. 2008).

There is an inherited predisposition to infection, and individuals with blood type O are more often infected, while blood types B and AB can confer partial protection against symptomatic infection. The reason for this protection remains obscured (Bucardo et al. 2009).

No specific treatment is available. Sanitizing of surfaces where the norovirus may be present is recommended. Moderate to severe cases require intravenous re-hydration.

Rotavirus

Rotavirus is the most common cause of acute nonbacterial gastroenteritis affecting approximately 130 million infants and children of up to 5 years with 600,000-800,000 deaths worldwide (Ball et al. 1996). It mainly occurs in winter months causing a life-threatening diarrhea in children younger than 2 years old. The infective dose is presumed to be 10-100 infectious viral particles. A person with rotavirus diarrhea often excretes far large numbers of virus than the infective particles (10^8-10^{10} infectious particles/ml of feces). These viruses are stable to the environment making environmental contamination inevitable, with a high risk of secondary infection in susceptible contacts through contaminated hands, objects, or utensils. Because of this, about 20% of the rotavirus infections diagnosed in pediatric hospitals are acquired in the hospital.

The virus infects mature enterocytes of the villous tip of the small intestine and causes diarrhea by producing an enterotoxin, the nonstructural rotavirus protein (NSP4), and by direct activation of the enteric nervous system. NSP4 causes diarrhea in various ways; firstly, impairs activities of intestinal Na^+-solute transport and inhibits water reabsorption by blocking the intestinal sodium/glucose cotransporter 1 (SC5A1), hence contributing to diarrhea (Halaihel et al. 2000); secondly, it impairs activities of intestinal disaccharidases leading to malabsorptive (Halaihel et al. 2000); and thirdly, it activates the enteric nervous system, producing an increased chloride secretory response through a calcium-dependent chloride secretory mechanism (Lundgren and Svensson 2000).

The rotavirus illness is a self-limiting disease characterized by vomiting, watery diarrhea, and low-grade fever. Children with severe cases usually require hospitalization and intravenous fluids. Death may occur due to severe dehydration. Rotavirus illness is generally mild in older children and adults because of acquired antibodies to the viruses. Asymptomatic cases do occur and serve an important transmission.

HIV-1

Although most diarrheas observed in HIV-patients are due to the opportunistic infections, HIV-1 can also cause severe watery diarrhea on its own. The mechanisms for this diarrhea relates to that of cholera toxin. It is mediated by the transactivating Tat peptide of HIV-1 whose role is two folds; first, it stimulates active fluid secretion in the intestinal epithelial cells (Berni Canani 2006); and second, it inhibits sodium ion and glucose transport activity, leading to osmotic diarrhea (Berni Canani 2006).

Parasites

Giardia Lamblia

Giardia lamblia is endemic and affects large populations of people worldwide. It is the most frequent cause of parasitic diarrhea in immunocompetent patients. In developed nations, *G. lambria* infects 2–5% of the population while in developing countries with poor sanitation and contaminated food or water sources, it may affect up to 20–30% of the population (Escobedo and Cimerman 2007).

Giardia organisms are often found in soil, food, and surfaces contaminated with feces containing infectious cysts. Infection follows ingestion of infective cysts acquired via person-to-person, water- and food-borne. As few as 10 to 25 cysts are competent to produce infection. Person-to-person transmission accounts for a majority of Giardia infections and is usually associated with poor hygiene and sanitation (Vesy and Peterson 1999; Baker 2007; Escobedo and Cimerman 2007). Water-borne transmission is through contaminated water supplies, such as water in rivers and lakes and improperly treated water that are reservoirs of the cysts. Often, contamination of surface water is caused by rain and wind carrying cysts from fields containing or fertilized by manures of infected humans, livestock, or wild animals to nearby rivers and streams (Baker 2007).

Following ingestion, *G. lamblia* cysts excyst to release trophozoites that adhere to the epithelium of the upper small intestine (mainly the duodenum) and damage the mucosal brush border without invasion (Hill 1990). The exact mechanism by which *G. lamblia* causes diarrhea remains obscured.

Symptoms usually begin 1 to 2 weeks after an individual becomes infected. In healthy individuals, symptoms may last 2 to 6 weeks. Symptoms include an abrupt onset of abdominal cramps, acute or chronic watery diarrhea, vomiting, foul flatus, and fever which may last for 3–4 days. In both the acute and insidious onsets of symptoms, stools become greasy and malodorous without blood or pus. There could be episodic diarrhea associated, at times, with steatorrhea and a malabsorption syndrome similar to celiac disease. The watery diarrhea may cycle with soft stools and constipation. Upper gastrointestinal symptoms including nausea, early satiety, bloating, substernal burning, egg-smelling halitosis, and acid indigestion may be exacerbated by eating and are generally present in the absence of soft stools. There could also be anorexia, malaise, fatigue, and weight loss in more than 50% of patients (Ortega and Adam 1997; Vesy and Peterson 1999; Baldi et al. 2009).

Treatment

In some patients the infection is cured spontaneously without treatment intervention. Recommended treatments for giardiasis are shown in Table 3.

Table 3. Treatments for Giardiasis

Medication	Adult dosage	Duration
First line of treatment		
Metronidazole (Flagyl)	250 mg p.o. t.d.s.	5 days
Tinidazole (Fasigyn)	2 g p.o.	Once
Nitazoxanide: Adult dosage:	500 mg b.i.d	3 days
Alternative treatment		
Paramomycin (Humatin)	25–35 mg/kg p.o. t.d.s.	7 days
Furazolidone (Furoxone)	100 mg p.o. q.d.s.	7-10 days
Quinacrine	100 mg p.o. t.d.s.	5 days
Albendazole (Albenza)	400 mg p.o. daily	5 days
Mebendazole (Vermox)	200–400 mg p.o. daily	5-10 days

Cryptosporidiosis

Cryptosporidiosis is a diarrheal disease caused by *Cryptosporidium* spp. The main causes of cryptosporidiosis in humans are *C. parvum* and *C. hominis*. However, *C. canis*, *C. felis*, *C. meleagridis*, and *C. muris* can also cause the disease in humans. The parasites are found throughout the world and during the past 2 decades, cryptosporidiosis has been recognized as one of the most common causes of waterborne disease in humans (Savioli et al. 2006; Davies and Chalmers 2009).

Cryptosporidium lives in the intestine of humans and animals. It completes its life cycle within a single host, resulting in oocysts which are excreted in feces. Infection follows ingestion of contaminated material such as earth, water, uncooked or cross-contaminated food that has been in contact with the feces of an infected individual or animal. As few as 2 to 10 oocysts can initiate an infection (Chen et al. 2003; Davies and Chalmers 2009). Ingested oocysts excyst in the small intestine and become located in the brush border of the small intestinal epithelial cells, mainly in the jejunum. It then attaches to an 85 kDa surface protein on intestinal epithelial cells via its apical glycoprotein CSL complex (Langer et al. 2001). When the organisms touch the epithelial membrane, the CSL complex envelops the parasite to make it intracellular but extracytoplasmic (Ryan et al. 2004). The parasite then induces fluid secretion via multiple mechanisms involving damage to the microvilli where it attaches, increased local levels of prostaglandins and the subsequent cAMP-mediated chloride secretion, inhibition of electroneutral sodium chloride and decreased water absorption by the villous cells (Simon et al. 1994; Guarino et al. 1995; Winn et al. 2006).

Cryptosporidiosis is typically an acute short-term infection but can become severe and non-resolving in children and immunocompromised individuals. Symptoms appear from 2-10 days after infection and last for up to two weeks, or in some cases, up to one month. There are 3 possible forms of the illness in immunocompetent individuals; asymptomatic, acute diarrhea, or persistent diarrhea lasting for a few weeks. Diarrhea is usually watery with mucushttp://en.wikipedia.org/wiki/Cryptosporidiosis-cite_note-Chen-4.

Additionally, there is often stomach pains or cramps, a low grade fever, nausea, vomiting, malabsorption, dehydration, anorexia, and weight loss (Chen et al. 2002; Ryan et al. 2004; Winn et al. 2006. About 60% of immunocompromised people (e.g. AIDS, neoplasia, and concurrent viral infection) may have persistent chronic watery diarrhea while 8% have a severe, cholera-like infection.

Treatment

A successful treatment for *Cryptosporidia* has not yet been found. Certain agents such as paromomycin, atovaquone, nitazoxanide, and azithromycin are sometimes used, but they usually have only temporary effects. Spiramycin and hyperimmune bovine colostrum are still under experimentation (Smith and Corcoran 2004). Effective treatment is primarily supportive. Oral and sometimes intravenous fluid replacement and lactose-free diet have been useful. For immunocompromised individuals, improving the immune status by probiotic *Saccharomyces boulardii* is helpful in managing cryptosporidium diarrhea (Ochoa et al. 2004).

Cyclospora Cayetanensis

Infection with *Cyclospora cayetanensis* is considered an emerging disease in developed but endemic in developing countries. The pathogen is similar to *Cryptosporidium* in both, morphology and the effects it causes in the small bowel mucosa. It is transmitted through ingestion of water or food contaminated with sporulated oocyst. The oocysts excyst in the gut releasing the sporozoites which proceed to invade the epithelial cells of the small intestine (Ortega et al. 1997)

Symptoms begin about 5-8 days following ingestion and may persist for a month or more. They include loose to watery diarrhea, nausea, vomiting, abdominal cramps, loss of appetite, weight loss; fever, chills, muscle aches, joint aches, generalized body aches, headache, or fatigue (Crist et al 2004).

Although it is thought to be self-limiting in immuno-competent individuals, cyclosporiasis can cause prolonged diarrhea that could be life threatening in immuno-compromised patients (Karanja et al. 2007).

Cyclosporiasis can be treated by trimethoprim-sulfamethoxazole at 160-800 mg b.i.d. p.o. for 7 days or 160-800 mg q.d.s. p.o. for 10 days in immunocompromised patients with AIDS.

Dientamoeba Fragilis

Until few years ago, *Dientamoeba fragilis* was considered a human commensal protozoan similar to *Entamoeba coli* and *Endolimax nana*. The parasite has emerged to be a cause of gastrointestinal disease with evidence of causing diarrhea (Norberg et al. 2003; Johnson et al. 2004; Stark et al. 2005). It affects people of all age but mostly young individuals below 24 years (Lagacé-Wiens et al. 2006). The parasite can be acquired through feco-oral transmission and via eggs of the pinworm, *Enterobius vermicularis* (Johnson et al. 2004; Lagacé-Wiens et al. 2006). The pathogenesis of the diarrhea is not yet known. Clinical symptoms include abdominal pain, cramping and a plethora of vague abdominal complaints.

D. fragilis infection can be treated with iodoquinol (650 mg, t.d.s. p.o. for 20 days) and doxycycline 100 (mg b.i.d. p.o. for 10 days). Other drugs include metronidazole, paromomycin, and secnidazole (Norberg et al. 2003; Johnson et al. 2004; Lagacé-Wiens et al. 2006).

Nonpathogenic Organisms

Diarrhea can be caused by organisms normally known to be non-pathogenic to the gut. The illness develops when the concentration the organisms is high. In most cases the symptoms are chronic abdominal discomfort and watery diarrhea. Examples include Candida spp and Blastocystis hominis (Gupta 1990; Suresh et al. 2009). Evidence is lacking to definitively implicate either of these organisms as causative agents of diarrhea

Inflammatory Diarrhea

In opposite to non-inflammatory diarrheal agents, the aetiological agents of inflammatory diarrheas target the large bowel, mainly the distal ileum and the colon. The organisms cause considerable acute intestinal inflammation and mucosal destruction by either secreting toxins or invading the epithelium (Giannella 2006; Navaneethan and Giannella 2008). The diarrhea presented by individuals infected with invasive organisms (e.g. *Shigella, Salmonella, Yersinia enterocolitica, Campylobacter jejuni, Enteroinvasive E. coli* (EIEC), and *Entamoeba histolytica*) will be bloody, mucoid, and with leucocytes or pus; there will be tenesmus, lower left quadrant abdominal pains; fever may follow invasion of the circulatory system. If the agents produce toxins without invading the epithelium, e.g. *Enterohemorrhagic E. coli* (EHEC), the patient will have watery diarrhea with or without blood, abdominal pains, and low grade fever.

Non-Invasive Inflammatory Diarrhea

Enteropathogenic E. Coli (EPEC)

The enteropathogenic *E. coli* (EPEC) is identified as causing attaching and effacing lesions on intestinal cells. The attachment of bacteria is made by shiga-like toxin. Following attachment, EPEC organisms are found in a close association with the intestinal mucosa (Donnenberg et al. 1997). In this association the organisms are closely associated with the apical surface of the epithelial cells, i.e. less than 20 nm separates the plasma membrane from the bacterium. The apical plasma membrane partly surrounds the attached organisms in a cup-like or pedestal-like extension on which the pathogens reside to ultimately cause severe disruption of the microvilli brush border. Disruption of the microvilli brush border is thought to be the prime cause of diarrhea (Fleckenstein and Kopecko 2001).

Enterohemorrhagic E. Coli (EHEC)

Enterohemorrhagic *E. coli* (EHEC) particularly causes a dangerous type of diarrhea. It is one of the most common causes of bloody diarrhea throughout the world (Navaneethan and Giannella 2008)

The disease is associated with food borne outbreaks traced to undercooked hamburger meat, unpasteurized apple juice or cider, salad, salami, and unpasteurized milk. Some outbreaks have also been traced to contaminated well water and improperly disinfected swimming pools. The illness develops following ingestion of the bacterium or preformed shiga toxin produced by hemorrhagic *E. coli* 0157:H7 and O26:H11 organisms (Griffin 2002). The ingested EHEC attach to the intestinal mucosa via a pilus. The attachment is followed by activation of protein kinase and intracellular release of calcium.

This process produces flattening and dissolution of villi, termed attaching–effacing lesions (Griffin 2002). In addition, EHEC secrete two shiga-like toxins; STX cytotoxins I and II (Su and Brandt 1995). The toxins are verocytotoxic and produce inflammation of the small intestine that leads to an initial nonbloody watery diarrhea. Later, the inflammation extends to involve the large intestine. Clinically, the diarrheal illness is designated as hemorrhagic colitis and is characterized by severe crampy abdominal pain and fever, followed within hours to one day by bloody diarrhea lasting five to seven days. Infection with EHEC can also cause extraintestinal lesions like hemolytic-uremic syndrome and thrombotic thrombocytopenic purpura (Griffin 2002).

Enteroaggregative *E. Coli* (EAEC)

Enteroaggregative *E. coli* (EAEC) are named so because they have fimbriae that aggregate tissue culture cells. They cause diarrhea by adhering to the epithelial brush border and altering cell function. Contrary to EPEC which produce localized adherence, EAEC produce a diffuse adherence in jejunal, ileal and colonic epithelium, with the latter being the principal target (Nataro and Kaper 1998). Adherence is mediated by the aggregative adherence fimbriae, particularly fimbria II (Okeke et al. 2000) while dispersal of EAEC and development of new foci of infection to cause diffuse adherence is via a protein dispersin (Sheikh et al. 2002). EAEC adherence stimulates mucus production and formation of a mucus biofilm, which might contribute to malnutrition and prolonged diarrhea (Vial PA et al. 1988). In addition, EAEC produce hemolysin and a heat stable enterotoxin (EAST1) similar to that of ETEC. The hemolysin and enterotoxin are linked with the development of acute inflammatory response and the associated enterocyte damage, cytokine release and intestinal secretion. The bacteria also trigger the host to produce IL-8 which attracts inflammatory cells and exacerbates further the epithelial cell destruction and fluid secretion (Huang et al. 2004). Being non-invasive, EAEC organisms cause watery diarrhea without fever. Occassionally, there can blood and mucus.

A closely related to EAEC is the diffusely adherent *E. coli* (DAEC) that causes a similar pathology and diarrhea but does not aggregate cells and its adherence pattern is more diffuse than that of EAEC.

Clostridium Difficile

Clostridium difficile causes pseudomembranous colitis which develops due to alteration of microbioata following uptake of broad-spectrum antibiotics such as clindamycin, cephalosporins and chinolonics. The antibiotics kill off competing microbioata in the intestine leaving behind bacteria with less competition for space and nutrients. The net effect is to permit much more extensive growth than normal of *Clostridium difficile*. By itself, *C. difficile* is an important nosocomial pathogen and the most frequently diagnosed cause of infectious hospital-acquired diarrhea (Hookman and Barkin 2007). It is acquired by the oral route from an environmental source or by contact with an infected person or a health care worker who serves as a vector.

The highly proliferating *C. difficile* produces UDP-glucose hydrolases and glucosyltransferases toxins A and B, which cause intense inflammation of the colonic mucosa with fluid and electrolyte secretion (Warny et al. 2005). Initially, the toxins attach to nonproteinaceous disaccharide galactose-β1–4-*N*-acetylglucosamine residues on colonic epithelial cells (Wilkins and Tucker 1989). The toxins then enter the enterocyte by endocytosis and catalyze the transfer of a glucose residue from UDP-glucose to guanosine-triphosphate-binding rhoproteins (Halaihel et al. 2000). The latter regulate cytoskeletal organization and gene expression. The end result of this signaling is disruption of protein synthesis and cell death (Warny and Kelly 2003) and activation of transcription factor NF-κB as well as MAP kinases and their subsequent inflammatory cytokine release (IL-1β, tumor necrosis factor, and IL-8). The inflammatory cytokines contribute to the marked intestinal inflammation and secretion following *C. difficile* infection (Giannella 2006).

The illness (pseudomembranous colitis) may occur months after antibiotic exposure, and may rarely occur without a past history of antibiotic use. It is characterized by offensive-smelling severe watery diarrhea, low-grade fever, abdominal pains and leukocytosis. The diarrhea is usually loose with a blood-streaked mucus and devastating with up to 30 bowel movements in a 24-hour period. It can be complicated by toxic megacolon, and can be fatal due to fluid loss, hypotension, and hypovolaemic shock.

Treatment is symptomatic. In many patients the problem is self-limiting and resolves following discontinuation of the antibiotic. In such patients no further therapy may be indicated. Otherwise, metronidazole 250-400 mg q 8 hours for 14 days in mild cases, and vancomycin 125 mg q 6 hours for 14 days in severe cases is advocated. However, due to expensiveness of vancomycin, the drug is often reserved for those patients who have experienced a relapse after a course of metronidazole. Adjunctive therapy may include cholestyramine that binds the toxin but does not eliminate the microorganism.

The probiotic *Saccharomyces boulardii* reduces the recurrence rate of pseudomembranous colitis.

Invasive Etiological Agents of Inflammatory Diarrhea

Shigella Dysenteriae

Shigella dysenteriae induces a superficial invasion of the intestinal mucosa. The organism is the most common cause of epidemic dysentery in condensed populations such as refugee camps, mental institutions, boarding schools or day-care centers. *S. sonnei* and *S. flexneri* also contribute to shigellosis but less common. Shigellosis is a major cause of diarrhea-related morbidity and mortality, especially in developing countries, with an estimated annual incidence of 165 million cases and 1 million deaths (Kotloff et al. 1999). The severity of the disease is variable depending on the underlying health of the individual as well as the infecting strain. Usually children, old, debilitated, or malnourished people are more severely affected. Among the three species, *S. sonnei* causes mild diarrhea.

Infection usually occurs through fecal-oral route by direct contact with contaminated objects or through ingestion of contaminated food or water. Occasionally, the housefly is a vector. Infection can be transmitted between people unless appropriate hygiene measures are undertaken. Some infected patients are asymptomatic and are those more likely to transmit infection to other people.

Shigella strains readily invade epithelial cells from the basolateral surface. They enter preferentially through M cells, which are specialized epithelial cells overlying lymphocyte-rich Peyer's patches. The invasion and the subsequent cell entry is a role of bacterial proteins IpaA, IpaB and IpaC secreted into the host cell membranes (Blocker et al. 1999) and the mammalian small GTPases Cdc42, Rac and Rho, which regulate the actin cytoskeleton. Injection of IpaA, IpaB and IpaC into the host cell membrane activates Cdc42, Rac (Van Nhieu et al. 1999) and Rho leading to depolymerization of actin filament and formation of membrane ruffles. Through membrane ruffling and macropinocytosis, *Shigella* organisms enter the colonic mucosa (Adam et al. 1995; Clerc and Sansonetti 1987). After engulfment, the pathogen rapidly lyses the surrounding vacuole and is released into the cytosol where it grows and divides (Sansonetti et al. 1986). The bacteria become coated with filamentous actin and begin to move through the cytoplasm leaving a trail of actin filaments behind that propels the bacterium (Bernardini et al. 1989; Zeile et al. 1996). In addition, the bacterium expresses *icsA* gene for production of IcsA membrane protein that hydrolyses ATP and directs the actin-based motility to the neighboring cell (Goldberg et al. 1993; Goldberg and Theriot 1995; Kocks et al. 1995). Pseudopodia containing bacteria trailed by actin are formed and engulfed by neighbouring cells, allowing *Shigella* to spread from cell to cell without contacting the extracellular milieu (Palmer et al. 1998). The bacterium then breaks out of the pseudopodia vacuoles and starts a new cycle of infection in this cell (Schesser et al. 1998).

From the enterocytes, *Shigella* organisms are able to spread to underlying macrophages. The infected macrophages undergo apoptosis and release infective bacteria and large quantities of the proinflammatory cytokines interleukin (IL)-1 and IL-8. Both apoptosis and cytokine release require the IpaB protein, independently of its role in bacterial cell entry. During the process, IpaB binds to caspase-1. The latter activates apoptosis and as a protease, cleaves pro-IL-1 into active IL-1. The produced IL-1 as well as the IL-8 attracts neutrophils into the intestinal lumen to cause the inflammation and epithelial cell destruction (Fleckenstein and Kopecko 2001). In addition, the neutrophils loosen the basolateral intercellular junctions increasing the cellular invasion by the organisms (Sansonetti et al. 1999).

In addition to the invasive mechanism, *Shigella* organisms also secrete an enterotoxin that inhibits protein synthesis causing cytotoxicity and cell death (Su C and Brandt 1995). The toxin also increases chloride secretion by stimulating intestinal secretion via upregulation of luminal galanin-1 receptors (Matkowskyj et al. 2000)

The onset of *Shigella* infection ranges from a day to a week but usually it takes two to four days after infection. Symptoms of *S. dysenteriae* and *S. flexneri* infection include multiple small-volume diarrheas with blood, mucous and pus in stool, fever, nausea, vomiting, stomach cramps, flatulence, rectal burning and straining during bowel movements (Echeverria et al 1999). Intestinal complications include perforation and severe protein loss. Extraintestinal complications include arthritis, hemolytic uremic syndrome, respiratory symptoms, meningismus, seizures and rashes.

Treatment of *S. dysenteriae* includes enteric precautions, low-residue diet and, most important, replacement of fluids and electrolytes with intravenous infusions of normal saline solution (with electrolytes) in sufficient quantities to maintain urine output of 40 to 50 ml/hour. Antibiotics are of questionable value but may be used in an attempt to eliminate the pathogen and thereby prevent further spread. Ampicillin 500 mg q.i.d., or co-trimoxazole 2 tablets b.i.d. for 5 days is the treatment of choice. Tetracycline can also be used. These antibiotics may be useful in severe cases, especially in children with overwhelming fluid and electrolyte loss. It is interesting to note that amoxicillin is not effective therapy for shigellosis. Sulfamethoxazole-trimethoprim and ciprofloxacin are also used to treat shigellosis. Antidiarrheals that slow intestinal motility are contraindicated because they delay fecal excretion of *S. dysenteriae* and prolong fever and diarrhea. At the moment, an investigational vaccine containing attenuated strains of *Shigella* appears promising in preventing shigellosis.

Enteroinvasive E. Coli (EIEC)

Similar to *Shigella*, Enteroinvasive *E. coli (EIEC)* causes a superficial mucosal invasion following consumption of contaminated food or water. The EIEC organisms are so closely related to *Shigella spp*. In fact, they both (*Shigella spp* and EIEC strains) belong to the species *E. coli* (Lan and Reeves 2002). Similar to Shigella, EIEC possess the virulence plasmid of about 220 kb and have ability to invade epithelial cells and disseminate from cell to cell. The organisms produce shiga-like toxin that enables penetration of the bacteria into the enterocytes to cause colitis via a mechanism similar to that of *Shigella spp*. Briefly, EIEC attach to M cells overlying lymphoid follicles, induce membrane ruffling, and enter the cells while within vacuole (Nhieu et al 2000). After entry, the bacteria rapidly lyse the vacuolar membrane to gain access to host cell cytoplasm, multiply within the cytoplasm, induce actin polymerization at one pole, and move through the cytoplasm to infect adjacent cells. The intracellular EIEC release peptidoglycans that are detected by the Nod 1 pathway which activates the transcription factor, nuclear factor kappa B, leading to production of proinflammatory cytokines like IL-8. The latter attracts neutrophils to the site of invasion to cause leading to inflammation (Girardin et al 2001, 2003). The EIEC are also capable of spreading to macrophages where they induce apoptosis and production of IL-1 to add onto the intestinal epithelial mucosal damage.

The EIEC disease may in some cases, resemble ischemia clinically, endoscopically and histologically. Like other enteroinvasive organisms, the clinical signs of EIEC include watery diarrhea, blood in stool, mucus in stool, abdominal cramps, vomiting, chills, malaise, fever, and abdominal pains

Yersinia Enterocolitica

Yersinia enterocolitica (and less commonly *Y. pseudotuberculosis*) is another invasive pathogen that produces an enterotoxin following penetration of intestinal epithelial cells. Its invasion is deeper than *Shigella* and EIEC as it reaches the intestinal submucosa. *Yersinia* is a frequent cause of bacterial gastroenteritis in children less than 5 years of age. The organism is found in the feces and lymph nodes of sick and healthy animals, including humans. It replicates at refrigerator temperatures and has been associated with contamination of blood and blood products. Infection follows consumption of contaminated meat, ice cream, and milk or water and mechanically from pet animals.

Yersinia organisms use the surface protein invasin to help breach the intestinal barrier early in the disease cycle. Within the deeper tissues, most of the organisms remain extracellular. The pathogenic ability of *Yersinia* centers at secretion systems that target effector molecules to host cells (Cornelis and Wolf-Watz 1997). In contrast to *Shigella* and *Salmonella*, which use these systems to gain entry into non-phagocytic cells, *Yersinia* uses this type of system to avoid uptake by phagocytic cells. This is via microinjection of about 12 bacterial effector proteins known as Yops into host cells. In the cell, YopH, YopT and YopE interact with specific host proteins to block the cytoskeletal changes required for bacterial uptake, thereby blocking the bacterial entry. Several additional Yops like YpkA, whose targets and activities are not yet known, are also delivered to host cells (Donnenberg 2000).

Macrophages infected with *Yersinia* undergo apoptosis induced by YopJ. This apoptosis seems to have a central role in the infection.

Symptoms of *Y. enterocolitica* range from simple gastroenteritis to invasive ileitis and colitis. There is fever, abdominal pain, bloody diarrhea, and diarrhea. The diarrheal illness is most frequently in children below 5 years of age. Older children develop mesenteric adenitis and associated ileitis, which mimic acute appendicitis. In adults the illness is an acute diarrheal episode that may be followed 2-3 weeks later by joint symptoms and a rash (erythema nodosum). Treatment is symptomatic. There is no evidence that antibiotics reverse the course of the gastrointestinal infection.

Campylobacter Jejuni

Similar to *Yersinia*, *Campylobacter jejuni* invades the epithelium up to the submucosa consumption of improperly cooked or contaminated foodstuffs or water. It may also be transmitted through close contact with a person experiencing diarrhea. It is more common than diarrhea from *Salmonella* and *Shigella* combined. *C. jejuni*-induced diarrhea results from an enterotoxin produced by the bacterium following attachment to the intestinal mucosa as well as entry of the bacterium into the intestinal mucosa. Either mechanism is capable of causing a moderate to severe intestinal inflammation with or without ulceration.

The enterotoxin produced by the bacterium is a nuclease called cytolethal distending toxin (CDT). It induces arrest of the cell cycle and DNA damage (Hickey et al 2000). *C. jejuni* invades the intestinal epithelium through the M cells underlying the Payer's patches and via a microtubule-based entry system (Oelschlaeger et al 1993). The invasion is followed by spread of the bacteria to adjacent cells by interacting with host invasion receptors located on the basolateral aspects of the enterocytes (Hu and Kopecko 2000).

The *C. jejuni* CDT, CDT-induced epithelial damage, and the bacterial invasion to intestinal mucosa trigger release of the chemokine IL-8 from the epithelium that attracts neutrophils into the intestinal mucosa to cause campylobacter enteritis or gastroenteritis. The resulting *C. jejuni* illness ranges from watery, noninflammatory diarrhea to acute inflammatory enterocolitis (Giannella 2006).

Signs and symptoms usually develop 2 to 4 days after exposure to the organisms, although symptoms can persist for a longer period (7-10 days), and relapses occur in as many as 25% of patients. Initially there is cramping, abdominal pain, nausea, vomiting, headache, and generalized malaise with or without fever. This is followed by a prolonged diarrheal illness with initial bloody diarrhea, slight improvement, and then increasing severity. Complications associated with campylobacteriosis include bacteremia, severe dehydration and electrolyte disturbances, Guillain-Barré syndrome, and Reiter's syndrome. Patients with campylobacteriosis who are immunocompromised are more susceptible to sepsis, endocarditis, meningitis, and thrombophlebitis because of the spread of the bacteria into the bloodstream.

Erythromycin 500 mg q.i.d. for 7 days is optimal therapy although it does not reduce the length of time that infected individuals shed the bacteria in their feces. Otherwise, most *C. jejuni* infections are self-limiting and are not treated with antibiotics.

Salmonella

Many types of *Salmonella* cause disease in both animals and people and the prevalence of different types of *Salmonella* species vary from country to country. However, the most common illness, enteritis, due to nontyphoidal *Salmonella* is food poisoning gastroenteritis caused mainly by serotypes *Salmonella enteritidis* and *S. typhimurium*. In the past two decades an antibiotic resistant strain *S. typhimurium* Definitive Type 104 (DT104) that first emerged in the United Kingdom in 1984, has added significantly to *Salmonella*-induced diarrheagenic illnesses in several parts of the world. In other countries like the United States, it is the second most prevalent strain (after *S. enteritidis*) of *Salmonella* found in humans. This strain poses a major new threat because it is resistant to several antibiotics normally used to treat people with *Salmonella* infections including ampicillin, chloramphenicol, streptomycin, sulfonamides, and tetracycline.

Salmonella organisms are widespread in the intestinal tracts of humans, birds, reptiles and other mammals. The organisms pass from the feces of these hosts to infect people or other animals. Thus *Salmonella* are usually transmitted to humans by eating inadequately processed foods or foods contaminated with animal feces. The organisms can survive for weeks in water, ice, sewage, or food. Contaminated foods usually look and smell normal. They are often of animal origin, such as beef, poultry, milk, or eggs, but all foods, including vegetables may become contaminated. Many raw foods of animal origin are frequently contaminated, but fortunately, thorough cooking kills *Salmonella*. Food may also become contaminated by the unwashed hands of an infected food handler, who forgot to wash his or her hands with soap after using the bathroom. In children younger than age 5, salmonellosis may occur from fecal-oral spread.

Following ingestion, the organisms penetrate and pass from gut lumen into epithelium of small intestine and the colon where they produce an enterotoxin similar to that of *Staphylococcus aureus*. This enterotoxin is responsible for the intestinal inflammation.

During invasion, *Salmonella* exploits the host cytoskeleton resulting in dramatic morphologic changes to the cell. The changes are mediated by the *Salmonella* pathogenicity island 1 (SPI1) that directs the uptake of the bacteria by non-phagocytic cells. The SPI1 secretory system includes homologues of the Ipa proteins of *Shigella* with similar, but not necessarily identical functions. Once *Salmonella* is in close contact with the epithelium, the bacterial SPI1 system secretes effector protein SopE that is microinjected into the host cell membrane. The SopE then activates host Rac and Cdc42 resulting in extensive membrane ruffling and the subsequent bacterial entry (Donnenberg 2000). The entire process occurs within minutes and when completed, *Salmonella* resides within membrane-bound vesicles, and the cytoskeleton returns to its normal distribution (Francis et al 1993). The latter is mediated by another bacterial protein, the SptP which is immediately secreted after entry. SptP acts directly on Rac and Cdc42 to antagonize the effects of SopE, and thereby returning the host cell to its normal state (Fu and Galán 1999).

The hallmark for *Salmonella* pathogenesis is survival and multiplication within macrophages. This is made possible by a second pathogenicity island, SPI2. Expression of the SPI2 secretion system is stimulated when the bacteria are inside macrophages. The secreted SPI2-encoded proteins are translocated into the host cell's cytosol and may have specific role. One such protein, SpiC, blocks vesicle trafficking and endosome fusion (Uchiya 1999) leading to failure of fusion of that phagosomes containing *Salmonella* with the lysosomes. As a result, the phagocyte is unable to deliver microbicidal compounds to the bacteria causing the bacteria to survive and replicate.

In addition to the invasion mechanism, *Salmonella* enterocolitis also results from the action of enterotoxins produced by the *Salmonella* and the outer-membrane lipopolysaccharide that contains the Vi antigen. Thus increased intestinal secretion results from both, the inflammatory reaction and the response to enterotoxin (Giannella et al 1972; Grassl and Finlay 2008).

Salmonella diarrheagenic illnesses are featured by sudden (12 to 36 hours after ingestion of contaminated foods) onset of symptoms, severe headaches, chills, nausea, vomiting, fever, flu-like symptoms, loss of appetite followed by abdominal cramps and diarrhea that lasts three to four days and then gradually subsides. These symptoms may persist for one to four days before subsiding. While most people recover successfully from salmonellosis, a few will experience long-term symptoms such as arthritis. The disease can be very serious or even fatal in individuals that are very young, elderly, or have weakened immune systems.

Treatment

Once an individual is infected with *Salmonella*, prolonged excretion can occur, particularly in children. Almost half of children younger than 5 years of age continue to shed *Salmonella* months after initial infection. In such patients, antibiotic therapy prolongs this excretion. It has been speculated that the administered antibiotics suppress the protective effects of intestinal microbioata paving way to continual survival and excretion of the *Salmonella*. In addition, it has been observed that antibiotics fail to reduce the clinical illness of *Salmonella*. Because of these observations, routine administration of antibiotics against salmonella gastroenteritis is generally contraindicated. Instead, uncomplicated cases are treated symptomatically. Patients with complicated salmonella gastroenteritis such as those with predisposing conditions or sepsis, or who are very young or very old should however be treated with ampicillin or co-trimoxazole.

Amebiasis

Amoebiasis, an acute and chronic disease caused by an intestinal protozoan parasite *Entamoeba histolytica*, is the second leading parasitic cause of death in humans after malaria (Baldi et al 2009). Globally, it infects about 50 million people annually and is responsible for 40,000–100,000 deaths a year (WHO 1997; Stanley 2003). Amoebiasis manifests from asymptomatic carrier state to a severe fulminating illness with intestinal mucosal inflammation and ulceration of the colon (Giannella 2006).

Most individuals get amoebiasis after ingestion of food or water contaminated with feces containing *E. histolytica* cysts. Unusual modes of transmission include oral and anal sex, and contaminated enema apparatus (van Hal et al 2007).

Following infection, *E. histolytica* trophozoites adhere to the colonic mucins and epithelial cells via its galactose–*N*-acetyl-[D]-galactosamine-inhibitable surface lectin (Ravdin and Guerrant 1981). After adhesion, channel-forming peptides called amebophores are formed that render the colonic cells immobile and losing their cytoplasmic granules, structures, and eventually their nuclei resulting in cytolysis (Ravdin et al 1980; Berninghausen and Leippe 1997). The trophozoites also disrupt the tight junction proteins causing a decrease in transepithelial resistance that leads to increased intestinal permeability. The parasite then invades the epithelial mucosa into the submucosal tissues to cause amoebic colitis. The invasion is triggered by contact between amoebic trophozoites and the extracellular matrix protein fibronectin, which triggers signaling cascades within the parasite, and causes actin rearrangements that alter adherence and motility (Meza 2000). In addition, *E. histolytica* trophozoites secrete cysteine proteinases encoded by six different genes (EhCP1 to EhCP6) that digest extracellular matrix proteins to facilitate trophozoite invasion by burrowing through colonic mucus and matrix proteins into and within the submucosal tissues (Que and Reed 2000). The host responds by production of inflammatory mediators and cells to cause a severe inflammation at the site of amoebic invasion. Through the mucosa and submucosal tissues, the *E. histolytica* trophozoites enter the portal circulation to the liver where they create their unique abscesses.

Clinical Presentation

In most *E. histolytica* infections, symptoms are absent or very mild and represent non-invasive disease. However, 4–10% of asymptomatic individuals infected with *E histolytica* develop disease over a year.

Patients with amoebic colitis present with a history of several weeks of gradual bloody and mucoid diarrhea, abdominal pain and tenderness. Multiple small volume mucoid stools are common, but profuse, watery diarrhoea might be noted. Because *E histolytica* invades the colonic mucosa, even if no blood is seen, stools are almost invariably haem-positive. Rectal bleeding without diarrhea may be seen, especially in children. White blood cells and pus depending on severity are visible in the stool. Fever is unusual (<40% of patients); weight loss and anorexia can be present. A fulminant or necrotizing amoebic colitis, with profuse bloody diarrhoea, fever, pronounced leucocytosis, widespread abdominal pain, and high mortality rate (40%) secondary to perforation may occur in 0.5% of patients (Stanley Jr 2003).

Some patients with amoebic liver-abscesses have concurrent amoebic colitis, though more often they have no bowel symptoms and their stool is usually negative for *E. histolytica* trophozoites and cysts. *Amoebiasis* may also cause urinary tract problems, genital disease (including rectovaginal fistulaes), perianal disease, and cutaneous lesions without bowel symptoms.

Treatment of Amoebiasis

When *E. histolytica* infection is confirmed, even if patients are asymptomatic, they should be treated to eliminate the organism and prevent further transmission. Advocated treatment is usually specific to the location of the disease. Therefore, therapeutic agents used to treat amebiasis act intraluminally, intramurally or systemically.

Asymptomatic carriages are solely treated with luminal amoebicide like oral paromomycin (Humatin) 500mg t.i.d. for 7 days; iodoquinol (Yodoxin) 650 mg t.i.d. for 20 days; or diloxanide furoate (Furamide) 500 mg t.i.d. for 10 days.

Symptomatic amoebiasis, including liver abscess, is treated with both tissue amoebicide and luminal amoebicide. This includes oral metronidazole 750–800 mg t.i.d. for 6–10 days (up to 14 days for liver abscess. However, because metronidazole is less effective against organisms within the bowel lumen, iodoquinol (650 mg t.i.d. for 20 days) must be added. Oral tinidazole 2 g o.p.d for 2-3 days (up to 7 days with liver abscess) and oral paromomycin 500 mg t.i.d. for 7 days are also effective (Stanley Jr 2003)

Chapter IV

Special Forms of Diarrhea

Traveler's Diarrhea

Traveler's diarrhea is characterized by an increase in frequency of unformed bowel movements, typically four to five loose stools in 24 hours, passed by a traveler. It is commonly accompanied by watery diarrhea, abdominal cramps, nausea, bloating, urgency, fever and malaise. Traveler's diarrhea usually begins abruptly, during travel or soon after returning home, and is generally self-limiting, lasting three to four days. Ten percent of cases persist longer than one week, approximately 2% longer than one month and very few beyond three months. It does not imply a specific organism, but ETEC is the most common causative agent (Levine et al 1993. The organisms adhere to the small intestine, where they multiply and produce an enterotoxin that causes fluid secretion and hence diarrhea.

Besides ETEC and other bacterial illnesses like *Salmonella* gastroenteritis and *Shigella* dysentery, a variety of viral and parasitic enteric pathogens are also potential causative agents of traveler's diarrhea (Table 4).

Treatment and Prevention of Traveler's Diarrhea

Most cases of traveler's diarrhea are mild and self-limited and the pathogen is most often not identified. As a result therapy should be considered optional. Recommended treatments for traveler's diarrhea are categorized as general, specific and prophylactic approaches.

Table 4. Pathogens implicated in travelers' diarrhea

Pathogen	Contribution to traveler's diarrhea
Enterotoxigenic *E. coli*	20-75%
Enteroaggregative *E. coli*	0-20%
Enteroinvasive *E. coli*	0-6%
Shigella spp	2-30%
Salmonella spp	0-33%
Campylobacter jejuni	3-17%
Vibrio parahemolyticus	0-31%
Aeromonas hydrophila	0-30%
Giardia lamblia	0-20%
Entamoeba histolytica	0-5%
Cryptosporidium sp	0-20%
Rotavirus	0-36%
Norovirus	0-10%

A. General

A general approach to avoid traveler's diarrhea is to use safe water, beverages and food. Travelers should maintain good hygiene when using water. This includes using safe water for drinking and teeth brushing, using safe bottled water only when one is sure that it has never been opened and re-sealed. Drinking water should be boiled for three to five minutes, filtered or treated with chloride bleach (2 drops per liter) or tincture of iodine (5 drops per liter). Beverages to drink should be safe like the bottled carbonated drinks and hot tea or coffee. An ultraviolet water purification device that allows people to quickly and conveniently treat small amounts of water, even in restaurant settings can be used by travelers. The device destroys bacteria and viruses' ability to live or replicate, it adds no taste to the water, allows the drinking of cold water, and is extremely economical compared with the cost of buying bottled water.

In case of acute attack, the traveler should drink oral rehydration solutions to replace lost fluids and electrolytes

All raw fruits and vegetables, raw meat and fish as well as meat or shellfish that is not hot when served, unrefrigerated food, and food from street vendors should be avoided. Unpasteurized milk or dairy products should not be ingested.

B. Specific

Travelers with acute attack can be given azithromycin or levofloxacin as single dose. Other antimicrobials and their prescription include diphenoxylate 1 tab, 2.5 mg after each bowel movement to maximum of 9 tab/day; loperamide 1 cap, 2.0 mg after each bowel movement to maximum of 8 cap/day; or Pepto-Bismol® 30 mL q 30 min, 8 doses. To decrease the severity of acute attack, co-trimoxazole 1 tab b.i.d. p.o. for 3 days or doxycycline 100 mg b.i.d. p.o. for 3 days can be used.

C. Prophylaxis

It is not recommended to take antimicrobials to prevent traveler's diarrhea because they kill off beneficial bacteria and create resistant breeds of pathogenic bacteria. However, for persons who are immunosuppressed or suffer chronic illness, co-trimoxazole 1 tab b.i.d. p.o. for days, doxycycline 100 mg b.i.d. p.o. for 3 days, or ciprofloxacin 500 mg b.i.d. p.o. for days are recommended. A combined use of bismuth subsalicylate and norfloxacin, ciprofloxacin, ofloxacin, or trimethoprim/sulfamethoxazole is also useful to prevent traveler's diarrhea. A vaccine, Dukoral, is given at one dose a few weeks before travel and another about a week before travel prevents traveler's diarrhea though not at 100% immunity.

It should be remembered that Traveler's diarrhea is fundamentally a sanitation failure, leading to bacterial contamination of drinking water and food. It is best prevented through proper water quality management systems as found in responsible hotels and resorts. In the absence of that, the next best option for travelers is to take precautions to prevent the disease:

Food Poisoning Diarrhea

In food poisoning syndrome, there is a brief but explosive diarrheal illness in subjects following ingestion of food contaminated with bacteria or bacterial toxins. Major bacteria for this syndrome include *Clostridium perfringens*, *Bacillus cereus*, *Staphylococcus aureus*, and *Salmonella* (Table 5). These bacteria account for nearly 90% of food poisoning outbreaks. In cases of ingestion of preformed toxins, diarrhea results from altered intestinal flux of salt and water in a similar way to enterotoxin-producing bacteria (Giannella 2006).

Table 5. Major food poisoning causing bacteria

Bacteria	Source	Symptoms	Therapy
Staphylococcus aureus	Ingestion of a preformed heat-stable, odorless and tasteless enterotoxin in poorly refrigerated desserts and seafoods	Nausea, vomiting, and profuse diarrhea within 4-8 hours	Spontaneous recovery within 24 hours. No specific therapy is available or necessary
Clostridium perfringens	Ingestion of a preformed toxin from spores that germinate in meats cooked to less than 50°C.	Diarrhea and crampy abdominal pain without vomiting within 8-24 hours	Spontaneous recovery within 24 hours. No specific therapy is available or necessary
Bacillus cereus	Ingestion of preformed toxin from cool unrefrigerated rice. Ingestion of the organism from meats, cereals, vegetables and milk	Vomiting syndrome. Diarrheal syndrome (profuse watery diarrhea). Other symptoms include nausea and dehydration	Both illnesses are short-lived. No specific therapy available or necessary
Salmonella	Ingestion of organism from poultry, pork, cattle, eggs, egg products, and milk	Diarrhea, fever, vomiting, abdominal cramps within 12-72 hours	Spontaneous recovery in 3-7 days. Symptomatic treatment and intravenous fluid. Antibiotics in severe cases

Chapter V

Treatment of Diarrhea

Diagnosis and Assessment

Treatment approach for diarrhea depends largely on classification of diarrhea (acute or chronic) and on understanding the main pathogenic mechanisms that resulted into the condition. Medical history and clinical evaluation of the patient as well stool examination are vital in deciding the treatment.

Physical examination of the patient is helpful in determining the severity of diarrhea and hydration status. A directed physical examination often leads to a more focused evaluation. Vital signs like temperature, pulse and blood pressure, and signs of volume depletion such as dry mucous membranes, decreased skin turgor, and confusion should be evaluated. Abdominal examination to assess the tenderness and distension should also be done. In addition, grossly bloody stool should be evaluated, while non-bloody stool should be tested for heme positivity.

While history and physical examination help to arrive to a diagnosis, specific diagnosis is needed if a more specific treatment of particular etiology is to be instituted. This should be carried out through fecal leukocyte determination, stool culture for enteric pathogens, stool examination for ova and parasites, and flexible sigmoidoscopy with biopsy.

In many cases where acute diarrhea can greatly affect the patient's life, therapy is prescribed before all diagnostic tests are exhausted (empirical therapy). It could involve rehydration and anti-microbial therapy. In patients where diagnosis is done, therapy is aimed at removing the causative agent as well as the diarrhea using anti-diarrheal agents (symptomatic therapy). The rational basis for empirical or symptomatic therapy stems on the inability of the intestine to reabsorb water.

Treatment

The principle components of the treatment of diarrhea are fluid and electrolyte replacement, dietary modifications, and drug therapy.

Fluid and Electrolyte Replacement

Most cases of acute diarrhea are typically self-limiting such that oral rehydration therapy (ORT) is central to the management. Its main goal is to prevent complications secondary to dehydration and its associated electrolyte disturbances and metabolic acidosis (Thapar and Sanderson 2004). This is done by oral rehydration salt (ORS) solutions which are effective on their own in ≥95% of cases of mild or moderate dehydration. They contain isotonic electrolytes and glucose or starch. Some of the ORS readily available are Pedialyte, Rehydrate, Ricelyte, Resol, and the WHO formula (Table 6). A homemade mixture of ½ teaspoon salt (3.5 g), 1 tsp baking soda (2.5 g $NaHCO_3$), 8 tsp sugar (40 g), and 8 oz (~230 ml) orange juice (1.5 g KCl), diluted to 1 L with water is as effective. If patients are otherwise health and are not dehydrated, adequate oral intake can be achieved with soft drinks, fruit juice, broth, soup and salted crackers. In cases of severe dehydration, or where oral rehydration is contraindicated or the patient is unable to drink, IV rehydration (e.g. with lactated Ringer's solution) may be required initially, with early reintroduction of ORT where possible (Dupont and Vernisse 2009). ORS are cheap and are able to be administered in many settings, including the home, making them advantageous over IV rehydration. Whether orally of IV administered, rehydration therapy has no effect on the duration of the disease or frequency of bowel motions, or the volume of stool. Hence, anti-diarrheal drugs intended to meet these needs are additionally used to treat the diarrhea.

Table 6. Some rehydration salt solutions and their composition

Solution	Carbohydrate (g/L)	Sodium mmol/L	Potassium
WHO 2002	14	75	20 mmol/L
CeraLyte 50	20	50	254 mg-1.5g/L
CeraLyte 70	40	70	1.5 g/L
Pedialyte	25	45	20 mmol/L
Enfalyte	30	50	25 mmol/L
Gatorade	45	20	3 mmol/L

Dietary Modifications

Osmotic diarrhea normally stops when the patient fasts. However, in most acute and infectious diarrheal illnesses, food abstinence is not recommended because foods provide calories necessary for renewal of enterocytes. Thus frequent uptake of fruit drinks, beverages, and soft easily digested foods like bananas, potatoes, and soups are recommended. Since some infections can cause transient lactase deficiency lactose containing dairy products should be avoided. Similarly, agents that increase intestinal motility like caffeinated beverages and alcohol should also be avoided.

Drug Therapy

Besides rehydration therapy, anti-diarrheal drugs are prescribed to reduce the frequency of bowel movements or the duration of illness which are not met by rehydration (Table 7). They function by inhibit intestinal motility (anti-motility agents), facilitate intestinal absorption (adsorbents), and inhibit intestinal secretion (anti-secretories).

Anti-motility agents known to inhibit intestinal peristalsis include agents that react with endogenous opiates such as B-endorphins. The B-endophins bind to mu receptors to block the gastrointestinal motility and stop diarrhea. Other anti-motility drugs include natural and synthetic opiates such as morphine, codeine, and loperamide. However, these natural and synthetic opiates have side effects of constipation and abdominal bloating. As such, they are generally ineffective as anti-diarrheal drugs. Adrenergic agonists, such as clonidine, which affect intestinal motility and transport, are also drugs of choice to treat diarrhea (Baldi et al 2009). In general terms, anti-motility drugs should be avoided in patients with fever, bloody diarrhea, and inflammatory diarrhea because they may prolong fever in shigellosis, toxic megacolon in *C. difficile* infection, and hemolytic-uremic syndrome in *E. coli* infections.

Table 7. Antidiarrheal drugs of choice

Class/Group	Drug	Dose	Mechanisms
µ-receptor agonists	Diphenoxylate	2.5-5 mg qid	Anti-motility
	Loperamide	2-4 mg qid	Anti-motility
	Codeine	15-60 mg qid	Anti-motility
	Morphine	2-20 mg qid	Anti-motility
Enkephalinase inhibitors δ-receptor	Racecadotril	1.5 mg/kg tid	Anti-secretory
Adrenergic agonists	Clonidine	0.1-0.3 mg tid	Anti-motility
Somatostatin analogue	Octreotide	30-250 µg tid	Anti-secretory
Bile acids binding substances	Cholestyramine	4-16 g/die	Adsorbent
Fibers	Psyllium	10-20 g/die	Adsorbent
Antisecretory salicylate	Bismuth subsalicylate	524 mg q ½ to 1 h	Anti-secretory
Antisecretory salicylate	Acetyl salicylic acid	325-650 mg q 4 h	Anti-secretory
Inhibitor of CFTR-mediated chloride secretion	SP 303 (Crofelemer)		Anti-secretory
Calmodulin inhibitors	Zaldaride	20 mg q 6 h for 2 days	Antisecretory
Serotonins	serotonin-3 (5-HT3)	Variable	Anti-motility

CFTR, Cystic fibrosis transmembrane conductance regulator.

Drugs that facilitate intestinal absorption include chelating agents, such as colestyramine, which are used with diarrhoea caused by bile acids, such as in post-cholecystechtomy or maldigestion syndromes; dietary food supplements, such as psyllium, which increase stool consistency and are useful for patients with incontinence; and diosmectite, which is a natural aluminomagnesium silicate clay. It gives strong adsorbent properties (Dupont and Vernisse 2009) that increase villous absorption to stop diarrhea.

Anti-secretory drugs advocated against diarrhea include endogenous opiates like enkephalins found in the intestinal epithelial cells. These opiates bind with delta receptors to reduce cAMP levels and thus reduce secretion of water and electrolytes. However, enkephalins are rapidly broken down by a specific enzyme, enkephalinase that determine their half-life. Enkephalinase inhibitors could be good antidiarrheal agents since they prolong the action of enkephalins. One such inhibitor is a recently developed drug, racecadotril, which is a potent anti-diarrheal agent proved to be purely an anti-secretory (Prado 2002; Wang et al 2005).

Other anti-diarrheal drugs may have mixed functions and additional functions like anti-pain or anti-microbial. Some include the endogenous opiate, dynorphins, which binds to kappa receptors to lower nociceptive sensitivity; somatostatin analogues, which are used in carcinoid syndrome or in other endocrinous diarrhoeas; and bismuth subsalicylate which reliefs diarrhea, nausea and abdominal pain;

Use of Antimicrobials

The use of antimicrobials may be indicated to patients with invasive organisms, traveler's diarrhea, immunosuppressed individuals, and the elderly. In these patients, empirical antibiotic treatment is warranted. In addition to the specific antimicrobials mentioned in the section on specific etiological agents of diarrhea, some of the antimicrobials used include fluoroquinolone, recommended in moderate illnesses; erythromycin or azithromycin for severe illness; and oral metronidazole and teicoplanin, which do not have adverse reaction to elderly patients (Thielman and Guerrant et al 2004; Nelson 2007). Antibiotic resistance and emergency of antimicrobial resistant strains and the killing of the gut microbioata together with its sequel as a result of continual use of anti-microbials is well understood by physicians. Prescribing these drugs should be done with caution if we are to win the battle against enteric pathogens.

Conclusion

Information about causes, mechanisms and effects of diarrhea has been accumulating in the past few years. This has opened new frontiers in pharmacological research in search of new and effective drugs to treat diarrhea. Together with hygienic support, the treatment of diarrheagenic illnesses in developed countries has resulted in significant decline in bacterial infections as opposes to developing countries where bacteria are the major cause of diarrhea. It seems however, that the hygienic conditions have contributed to the increase in the viral diarrhea in developed countries, where they form the major cause of diarrhea. Other factors like increased homosexuality in men, poverty and unhygienic conditions in developing countries, traveling of people from developed countries to tropical countries, use of antibiotics and emergency of antibiotic resistant organisms, hospitalization and nosocomial transmission in children, pose a big challenge to combating diarrhea, especially infectious diarrhea. This is exacerbated further by our suboptimal understanding of pathogenic mechanisms of some pathogens; and worse, their newly acquired factors for adaptability against chemotherapeutics. While rehydration therapy remains to be the recommended mainstay of treatment for diarrhea, designing and developing adjunct antidiarrheal agents aimed at reducing the stool volume and frequency of the bowel as well as antimicrobials to eliminate infectious agents, is still an area of further intense studies. The studies may focus on counteracting the side effects of these drugs as well as developing new drugs that are more effective. The discovery of the anti-secretory racecadotril is, at the present, one of such successful researches. Indeed, as more causes of diarrhea and other immunosuppressive diseases emerge, we must be braced to design new therapeutic approaches against diarrhea in addition to rehydration.

References

Adam, T; Arpin, M; Prevost, MC; Gounon, P; Sansonetti, PJ. Cytoskeletal rearrangement and the functional role of T-plastin during entry of *Shigella flexneri* into HeLa cells. *J. Cell Biol.* 1995 129, 367-381.

Agata, N; Ohta, M; Arakawa, Y; Mori, M. The bceT gene of Bacillus cereus encodes an enterotoxic protein. *Microbiol.* 1995 141, 983-988.

Alam, NH; Ashraf, H. Treatment of infectious diarrhea in children. *Pediatr. Drugs.* 2003 5, 151-165

Anderson, EJ; Weber, SG. Rotavirus infection in adults. *Lancet Infect. Dis.* 2004 4, 91–99.

Arnesen, LPS; Fagerlund, A; Granum, PE. Fromsoil to gut: Bacillus cereus and its food poisoning toxins. *FEMS Microbiol. Rev.* 2008 32, 579–606.

Asha, NJ; Tompkins, D; Wilcox, MH. Comparative analysis of prevalence, risk factors, and molecular epidemiology of antibiotic-associated diarrhea due to *Clostridium difficile, Clostridium perfringens*, and *Staphylococcus aureus. J. Clin. Microbiol.* 2006 44, 2785-2791.

Baker, J.R. Advances in Parasitology. *Elsevier Science & Technology Books.* p. 131, 2007.

Baldi, F; Bianco, MA; Nardone, G; Pilotto, A; Zamparo E. Focus on acute diarrhoeal disease. *World J. Gastroenterol.* 2009 15, 3341-3348

Ball, JM; Tian, P; Zeng, CQ; Morris, AP; Estes, M. Age-dependent diarrhea induced by a rotaviral nonstructural glycoprotein. *Science.* 1996 272, 101-104

Beecher, DJ; Schoeni, JL; Wong, AC. Enterotoxic activity of hemolysin BL from *Bacillus cereus. Infect. Immun.* 1995 63, 4423–4428.

Bernardini, ML; Mounier, J; d'Hauteville, H; Coquis-Rondon, M; Sansonetti, PJ. Identification of icsA, a plasmid locus of Shigella flexneri that governs bacterial intra-and intercellular spread through interaction with F-actin. *Proc. Natl. Acad. Sci. U. S. A.* 1989;86:3867-71.

Berni Canani, R. Inhibitory effect of HIV-1 Tat protein on the sodium-D-glucose symporter of human intestinal epithelial cells. *AIDS.* 2006 20, 5-10

Berninghausen, O; Leippe, M. Necrosis versus apoptosis as the mechanism of target cell death induced by *Entamoeba histolytica*. *Infect. Immun.* 1997 65, 3615–3621.

Binder, HJ. Mechanisms underlying the absorption of water and ions. *Int. Rev. Physio.l* 1977 12, 285-304.

Blocker, A; Gounon, P; Larquet, E; Niebuhr, K; Cabiaux, V; Parsot, C; Sansonetti, P. The tripartite type III secreton of *Shigella flexneri* inserts IpaB and IpaC into host membranes. *J. Cell Biol.* 1999 147, 683–693

Boyce, JM; Havill, NL. Nosocomial antibiotic-associated diarrhea associated with enterotoxin-producing strains of methicillin-resistant Staphylococcus aureus. *Am. J. Gastroenterol.* 2005 100: 1828–1834.

Bucardo, F; Kindberg, E; Paniagua, M; Grahn, A; Larson, G; Vildevall, M; Svensson, L. Genetic susceptibility to symptomatic norovirus infection in Nicaragua. *J. Med. Virol.* 2009 81, 728-735.

Cabello, FC; Espejo, R; Hernandez, MC; Rioseco, ML; Ulloa, J; Vergara, JA. Vibrio parahaemolyticus O3:K6 Epidemic Diarrhea, Chile, 2005 *Emerg. Infect. Dis.* 2007 13, 655–656

Carvalho-Costa, FA; Goncalves, AQ; Lassance, SL; de Albuquerque, CP; Leite, JP; B´ oia, MN. Detection of *Cryptosporidium* spp and other intestinal parasites in children with acute diarrhea and severe dehydration in Rio de Janeiro. *Rev. Soc. Bras. Med. Trop.* 2007 40, 346–348.

Chen, W; Harp, JA; Harmsen, AG. *Cryptosporidium parvum* infection in gene-targeted B cell-deficient mice. *J. Parasitol.* 2003 89, 391–393.

Chen, XM; Keithly, JS; Paya, CV; LaRusso, NF. Cryptosporidiosis. *N Engl. J. Med. 2002* 346, 1723–1731

Ciarlet, M; Estes, MK. Rotavirus and calicivirus infections of the GI tract. *Curr. Opin. Gastroenterol.* 2001 17, 10–16.

Clerc, P; Sansonetti, PJ. Entry of *Shigella flexneri* into HeLa cells: evidence for directed phagocytosis involving actin polymerization and myosin accumulation. *Infect. Immun.* 1987 55 2681-2688.

Cornelis, GR; Wolf-Watz, H. The *Yersinia* Yop virulon: a bacterial system for subverting eukaryotic cells. *Mol. Microbiol.* 1997 23, 861–867.

Crist, A; Morningstar, C; Chambers, R; Fitzgerald, T; Stoops, D; Deffley, M. Outbreak of cyclosporiasis associated with snow peas — Pennsylvania, 2004. *MMWR.* 2004 53, 876-878.

Davies, AP; Chalmers RM. Cryptosporidiosis. *BMJ.* 2009 339, b4168

Dittmar, E; Beyer, P; Fischer, D; Sch"afer, V; Schoepe, H; Bauer, K; Schlösser, R. Necrotizing enterocolitis of the neonate with *Clostridium perfringens*: diagnosis, clinical course, and role of alpha toxin. *Eur. J. Pediatr.* 2008, 167, 891-895.

Donnenberg, MS. Pathogenic strategies of enteric bacteria. *Nature.* 2000 406, 768-774

Donnenberg, MS; Kaper, JB; Finlay, BB. Interactions between enteropathogenic *Escherichia coli* and host epithelial cells. *Trends Microbiol.* 1997 5, 109–114

Donskey, CJ. The role of the intestinal tract as a source for transmission of nosocomial pathogens. *Curr. Infect. Dis. Rep.* 2004 6, 420–425.

Dupont, C; Vernisse, B. Anti-diarrheal effects of diosmectite in the treatment of acute diarrhea in children *Pediatr. Drugs.* 2009 11, 89-99

Echeverria, P; Sethabutr, O; Pitarangsi, C. Microbiology and diagnosis of infections with Shigella and enteroinvasive Escherichia coli. *Rev. Infect. Dis.* 1991 13 Suppl 4, S220-S225

Edmonds, CJ. Absorption and secretion of fluid and electrolytes by the rectum. *Scand. J. Gastroenterol.* 1984 Suppl. 93, 79-87

Ehling-Schulz, M; Fricker, M; Scherer, S. Bacillus cereus, the causative agent of an emetic type of food-borne illness. *Mol. Nutr. Food Res.* 2004 48, 479–487.

Escobedo, AA; Cimerman, S. Giardiasis: a pharmacotherapy review. *Expert. Opin. Pharmacother.* 2007 8, 1885-1902

Evans, DG; Silver, RP; Evans, DJ Jr, Chase, DG; Gorbach, SL. Plasmid-controlled colonization factor associated with virulence in *Escherichia coli* enterotoxigenic for humans. *Infect. Immun.* 1975 12, 656–667

Fagerlund, A; Lindb"ack, T; Storset, AK; Granum, PE; Hardy, SP. *Bacillus cereus* Nhe is a pore-forming toxin with structural and functional properties similar to the ClyA (HlyE, SheA) family of haemolysins, able to induce osmotic lysis in epithelia. *Microbiology.* 2008 154, 693–704.

Field M. Intestinal ion transport and the pathophysiology of diarrhea. *J. Clin. Invest.* 2003 111, 931-943

Fine, KD; Santa Ana, CA; Fordtran, JS. Diagnosis of magnesium-induced diarrhea. *N. Engl. J. Med.* 1991 324, 1012-1017.

Fleckenstein, JM; Kopecko, DJ. Breaching the mucosal barrier by stealth: an emerging pathogenic mechanism for enteroadherent bacterial pathogens. *J. Clin. Invest.* 2001 107, 27-30.

Fleckenstein, JM; Kopecko, DJ. Breaching the mucosal barrier by stealth: an emerging pathogenic mechanism for enteroadherent bacterial pathogens. *J. Clin. Invest.* 2001 107, 27–30

Flemming, K; Ackermann, G. Prevalence of enterotoxin producing *Staphylococcus aureus* in stools of patients with nosocomial diarrhea. *Infection.* 2007 35, 356-358.

Fordtran, JS; Rector, FC Jr; Carter, NW. The mechanisms of sodium absorption in the human small intestine. *J. Clin. Invest.* 1968 47, 884-900.

Francis, CL; Ryan, TA; Jones, BD; Smith, SJ; Falkow, S. Ruffles induced by *Salmonella* and other stimuli direct macropinocytosis of bacteria. *Nature.* 1993 364, 639-642.

Fu, YX; Galán, JE. A *Salmonella* protein antagonizes Rac-1 and Cdc42 to mediate host-cell

Giannella RA (2006) Infectious enteritis and proctocolitis and food poisoning. In: *Sleisenger & Fordtran's Gastrointestinal and Liver Disease*, edn 8 2333–2391 (Ed. Feldman M) Philadelphia: WB Saunders

Girardin, SE; Boneca, IG; Carneiro, LAM. Nod1 detects a unique muropeptide from Gram-negative bacterial peptidoglycan. *Science.* 2003 300, 1584–1587.

Girardin, SE; Tournebize, R; Mavris, M. CARD4/Nod1 mediates NF-kappa B and JNK activation by invasive *Shigella flexneri*. *EMBO Rep.* 2001 2, 736–742.

Goldberg, MB; Barzu, O; Parsot, C; Sansonetti, PJ. Unipolar localization and ATPase activity of IcsA, a Shigella flexneri protein protein involved in intercellular movement. *Infectious Agents Dispatch.* 1993 2, 210-211.

Goldberg, MB; Theriot, JA. *Shigella flexneri* surface protein IcsA is sufficient to direct actin-based motility. *Proc. Natl. Acad. Sci. U. S. A.* 1995 92, 6572-6576.

Grabitske, HA; Slavin, JL. Gastrointestinal effects of low-digestible carbohydrates. *Crit. Rev. Food Sci. Nutr.* 2009 49, 327-360.

Granum, PE. *Bacillus cereus* and its toxins. *J. Appl. Bacteriol. Symp.* 1994 Suppl 76, 61S-66S.

Granum, PE. *Clostridium perfringens* toxins involved in food poisoning. *Int. J. Food Microbiol.* 1990 10, 101–112.

Grassl, GA; Finlay, BB. Pathogenesis of enteric *Salmonella* infections. *Curr. Opin. Gastroenterol.* 2008 24, 22–26.

Gravet, A; Rondeau, M; Harf-Monteil, C; Grunenberger, F; Monteil, H; Scheftel, JM; Prevost, G. Predominant *Staphylococcus aureus* isolated from antibioticassociated diarrhea is clinically relevant and produces enterotoxin A and the bicomponent toxin LukE lukD. *J. Clin. Microbiol.* 1999 37, 4012-4019.

Griffin PM. *Escherichia coli* O157:H7 and other enterohemorrhagic *E. coli*. In *Infections of the GI Tract,* edn 2 627–642 (Eds Blaser M) Philadelphia: Lippincott Williams & Wilkins, 2002.

Guarino, A; Canani, RB; Casola, A; Pozio, E; Russo, R; Bruzzese, E; Fontana, M; Rubino, A. Human intestinal cryptosporidiosis: secretory diarrhea and enterotoxic activity in Caco-2 cells. *J. Infect. Dis.* 1995 171, 976-983

Halaihel, N; Lievin, V; Alvarado, F; Vasseur, M. Rotavirus infection impairs intestinal brush-border membrane Na (+) solute co-transport activities in young rabbits. *Am. J. Physiol. Gastrointest. Liver Physiol.* 2000 279, G587-G596

Hally, RJ; Rubin, RA; Fraimow, HS; Hoffman-Terry, ML. Fatal *Vibrio parahemolyticus* septicemia in a patient with cirrhosis. A case report and review of the literature. *Dig. Dis. Sci.* 1995 40, 1257-1260.

He, T; Venema, K; Priebe, MG; Welling, GW; Brummer, RJ; Vonk, RJ. The role of colonic metabolism in lactose intolerance. *Eur. J. Clin. Invest.* 2008 38, 541-547

Hersh, D; Monack, DM; Smith, MR; Ghori, N; Falkow, S; Zychlinsky, A. The *Salmonella* invasin SipB induces macrophage apoptosis by binding to caspase-1. *Proc. Natl. Acad. Sci. U.S.A.* 1999 96, 2396–2401

Hickey, TE; McVeigh, AL; Scott, DA; Michielutti, RE; Bixby, A; Carroll, SA; Bourgeois, AL; Guerry, P. *Campylobacter jejuni* cytolethal distending toxin mediates release of interleukin-8 from intestinal epithelial cells. *Infect. Immun.* 2000 68: 6535–6541

Hill DR (1990) *Giardia lamblia*. In: *Principles and Practice of Infectious Diseases* 2487-2493 (Eds Mandell GL *et al.*) Philadelphia: Churchill Livingstone.

Holmberg, SD; Blake, PA. Staphylococcal food poisoning in the United States. New facts and old misconceptions. *JAMA.* 1984 251, 487–489.

Hookman, P; Barkin, JS. Review: Clostridium difficile associated disorders/diarrhea and Clostridium difficile colitis: the emergence of a more virulent era. *Dig. Dis. Sci.* 2007 52, 1071-1075

Hu, L; Kopecko, DJ. (2000) Interactions of *Campylobacter* with eukaryotic cells: gut luminal colonization and mucosal invasion mechanisms. In

Campylobacter, edn 2 191–205 (Eds Nachamkin I and Blaser MJ) Washington, DC: ASM Press

Huang, DB; Okhuysen, PC; Jiang, ZD; DuPont, HL. Enteroaggregative *Escherichia coli*: an emerging enteric pathogen. *Am. J. Gastroenterol.* 2004 99, 383-389

Johnson, EH; Windsor, JJ; Clark, CG. Emerging from obscurity: biological, clinical, and diagnostic aspects of *Dientamoeba fragilis*. *Clin. Microbiol. Rev.* 2004 17, 553-570.

Johnston, D; Holdsworth, PJ; Smith, AH. Preservation of ileocecal junction and entire anal canal in surgery for ulcerative colitis--a "two-sphincter" operation. *Dis. Colon Rectum.* 1989 32, 555-561.

Jolivet-Reynaud, C; Popoff, MR; Vinit, MA; Ravisse, P; Moreau, H; Alouf, JE. Enteropathogenicity of Clostridium perfringens b-toxin and other clostridial toxins. *Zb. Bacteriol. Microbiol. Hyg.* 1986 Suppl 15, 145–151.

Karanja, RM; Gatei, W; Wamae, N. Cyclosporiasis: an emerging public health concern around the world and in Africa. *African Health Sciences.* 2007 7, 62-67

Kocks, C; Marchand, JB; Gouin, E; d'Hauteville, H; Sansonetti, PJ. The unrelated surface proteins ActA of Listeria monocytogenes and IcsA of Shigella flexneri are sufficient to confer actin-based motility on Listeria innocua and Escherichia coli respectively. *Mol. Microbiol.* 1995 18, 413-423.

Kotloff, KL; Winickoff, JP; Ivanoff, B; Clemens, JD; Swerdlow, DL; Sansonetti, PJ; Adak, GK; Levine, MM; Global burden of Shigella infections: implications for vaccine development and implementation of control strategies. *Bull. World Health Organ.* 1999 77, 651-666

Labbé, RG. 2000. Clostridium perfringens. In: Lund, B., Baird-Parker, T., Gould, G. (Eds.), *The Microbiological Safety and Quality of Food.* Aspen Publishers, MD, USA, pp. 1110–1135.

Lagacé-Wiens, PR; VanCaeseele, PG; Koschik, C. *Dientamoeba fragilis*: an emerging role in intestinal disease. *CMAJ.* 2006 175, 468-469

Lan, RT; Reeves, PR. Escherichia coli in disguise: molecular origins of *Shigella*. *Microb. Infect.* 2002 4, 1125–1132.

Langer, RC; Schaefer, DA; Riggs, MW. Characterization of an intestinal epithelial cell receptor recognized by the *Cryptosporidium parvum* sporozoite ligand CSL. *Infect. Immun.* 2001 69, 1661-1670

Layer, P; von der Ohe, MR; Holst, JJ; Jansen, JB; Grandt, D; Holtmann, G; Goebell, H. Altered postprandial motility in chronic pancreatitis: role of malabsorption. *Gastroenterology.* 1997 112, 1624–1634.

Levine, MM; Ferreccio, C; Prado, V; Cayazzo, M; Abrego, P; Martinez, J; Maggi, L; Baldini, MM; Martin, W; Maneval, D. Epidemiologic studies of *Escherichia coli* diarrheal infections in a low socioeconomic level periurban community in Santiago, Chile. *Am. J. Epidemiol.* 1993 138, 849–869

Lindberg, E; Nowrouzian, F; Adlerberth, I; Wold, AE. Longtime persistence of superantigen-producing *Staphylococcus aureus* strains in the intestinal microflora of healthy infants. *Pediatr. Res.* 2000 48, 741–747.

Lis, E; Korzekwa, K; Bystroń, J; Żarczyńska, A; Dabrowska, A; Molenda, J; Bania, J. Enterotoxin gene content in *Staphylococcus aureus* from the human intestinal tract. *FEMS Microbiol. Lett.* 2009 296, 72–77.

Lund, T; De Buyser, ML; Granum, PE. A new cytotoxin from *Bacillus cereus* that may cause necrotic enteritis. *Mol. Microbiol.* 2000 38, 254–261.

Lund, T; Granum, PE. Characterisation of a nonhaemolytic enterotoxin complex from *Bacillus cereus* isolated after a foodborne outbreak. *FEMS Microbiol. Lett.* 1996 141, 151–156.

Lundgren, O; Svensson, L. Pathogenesis of Rotavirus diarrhea. *Microbes Infect.* 2001 3, 1145-1156

Malago, JJ; Koninkx, JFJG; Douma, PM; Dirkzwager, A; Veldman, A; Hendriks, HGCJM; van Dijk, JE. Differential modulation of enterocyte-like Caco-2 cells after exposure to short chain fatty acids. *Food Additives and Contaminants.* 2003 20, 427-437.

Marcos, LA; DuPont, HL. Advances in defining etiology and new therapeutic approaches in acute diarrhea. *J. Infect.* 2007 55, 385-393

Matkowskyj, KA; Danilkovich, A; Marrero, J; Savkovic, SD; Hecht, G; Benya, RV. Galanin-1 receptor upregulation mediates the excess colonic fluid production caused by infection with enteric pathogens. *Nat. Med.* 2000 6: 1048–1051.

Metz, DC. Diagnosis of non-Zollinger-Ellison syndrome, non-carcinoid syndrome, enteropancreatic neuroendocrine tumours. *Ital. J. Gastroenterol. Hepatol.* 1999 31, Suppl 2, S153-159.

Meza I. Extracellular matrix-induced signaling in *Entamoeba histolytica*: its role in invasiveness. *Parasitol. Today.* 2000 16, 23–28.

Moss, J; Richardson, SH. Activation of adenylate cyclase by heat-labile *E. coli* enterotoxin. *J. Clin. Invest.* 1978 62, 281–285.

Mourad, FH; O'Donnell, LJ; Dias, JA; Ogutu, E; Andre, EA; Turvill, JL; Farthing, MJ. Role of 5-hydroxytryptamine type 3 receptors in rat intestinal fluid and electrolyte secretion induced by cholera and *Escherichia coli* enterotoxins. *Gut.* 1995 37, 340–345.

Musher, DM; Musher, BL. Contagious acute gastrointestinal infections. *N. Engl. J. Med.* 2004 351, 2417-2427

Naik, S; Smith, F; Ho, J; Croft, NM; Domizio, P; Price, E; Sanderson, IR; Meadows, NJ. Staphylococcal enterotoxins G and I, a cause of severe but reversible neonatal enteropathy. *Clin. Gastroenterol.* 2008 H 6, 251–254.

Nakagomi, T; Correia, JB; Nakagomi, O; Montenegro, FM; Cuevas, LE; Cunliffe, NA; Hart, CA. Norovirus infection among children with acute gastroenteritis in Racife, Brazil: disease severity is comparable to rotavirus gastroenteritis. *Arch. Virol.* 2008 153, 957-960.

Nasmyth, DG; Williams, NS. Pressure characteristics of the human ileocecal region--a key to its function. *Gastroenterology.* 1985 89, 345-351

Nataro, JP; Kaper, JB. Diarrheaegenic *E. coli. Clin. Microbiol. Rev.* 1998 11, 142-201

Navaneethan, U; Giannella, RA. Mechanisms of infectious diarrhea. *Nat. Clin. Pract. Gastroenterol. Hepatol.* 2008 5, 637-647.

Nelson R. Antibiotic treatment for Clostridium difficileassociated diarrhea in adults. *Cochrane Database Syst. Rev.* 2007

Norberg, A; Nord, CE; Evengard, B. *Dientamoeba fragilis* - a protozoal infection which may cause severe bowel distress. *Clin. Microbiol. Infect.* 2003 9, 65-68.

Ochoa, TJ; Salazar-Lindo, E; Cleary, TG. Management of children with infection-associated persistent diarrhea. *Semin. Pediatr. Infect. Dis.* 2004 15, 229–236.

Oelschlaeger, TA; Guerry, P; Kopecko, DJ. Unusual microtubuledependent endocytosis mechanisms triggered by *Campylobacter jejuni* and *Citrobacter freundii. Proc. Natl. Acad. Sci. U.S.A.* 1993 90, 6884–6888

Okeke, IN; Lamikanra, A; Czeczulin, J; Dubovsky, F; Kaper, JB; Nataro, JP. Heterogeneous virulence of enteroaggregative *Escherichia coli* strains isolated from children in Southwest Nigeria. *J. Infect. Dis.* 2000 181, 252-260

Oku, T; Hongo, R; Nakamura, S. Suppressive effect of cellulose on osmotic diarrhea caused by maltitol in healthy female subjects. *J. Nutr. Sci. Vitaminol. (Tokyo)* 2008 54, 309-314.

Ortega, Y; Nagle, R; Gilman, RH; Watanabe, J; Miyagui, J; Kanugusuku, P. Pathologic and clinical findings in patients with cyclosporiasis and a description of intracellular parasite life-cycle stages. *J. Infect. Dis.* 1997 176, 1584-1589.

Ortega, YR; Adam, RD. Giardia: overview and update. *Clin. Infect. Dis.* 1997 25, 545-549

Palmer, LE; Hobbie, S; Galán, JE; Bliska, JB. YopJ of *Yersinia pseudotuberculosis* is required for the inhibition of macrophage TNF-a production and downregulation of the MAP kinases p38 and JNK. *Mol. Microbiol.* 1998 27, 953–965.

Pezzilli, R. Chronic pancreatitis: Maldigestion, intestinal ecology and intestinal inflammation. *World J. Gastroenterol.* 2009 15, 1673-1676.

Prado, D. A multinational comparison of racecadotril and loperamide in the treatment of acute watery diarrhoea in adults. *Scand. J. Gastroenterol.* 2002 37, 656-661

Que X, Reed SL. Cysteine proteinases and the pathogenesis of amebiasis. *Clin. Microbiol. Rev.* 2000 13, 196–206.

Quiqley, EM; Phillips SF. The ileocecal (ileocolonic) sphincter. *Z. Gastroenterol.* 1983 21, 47-55

Ratnaike RN, Jones TE. Mechanisms of drug-induced diarrhoea in the elderly. *Drugs Aging.* 1998; 13: 245-253

Ravdin JI, Croft BY, Guerrant RL. Cytopathogenic mechanisms of *Entamoeba histolytica*. *J. Exp. Med.* 1980 152, 377–390.

Ravdin, JI; Guerrant, RL. Role of adherence in cytopathogenic mechanisms of *Entamoeba histolytica*: study with mammalian tissue culture cells and human erythrocytes. *J. Clin. Invest.* 1981 68, 1305–1313

Ray, AJ; Pultz, NJ; Bhalla, A; Aron, DC; Donskey, CJ. Coexistence of vancomycin-resistant enterococci and Staphylococcus aureus in the intestinal tracts of hospitalized patients. *Clin. Infect. Dis.* 2003 37, 875–881.

Rood, JI; Cole, ST. Molecular genetics and pathogenesis of *Clostridium perfringens*. *Microbiol. Rev.* 1991 55, 621-648.

Russo, MA; Högenauer, C; Coates, Jr, SW; Santa Ana, CA; Porter, JL; Rosenblatt, RL; Emmett, M; Fordtran, JS. Abnormal passive chloride absorption in cystic fibrosis jejunum functionally opposes the classic chloride secretory defect. *J. Clin. Invest.* 2003 112, 118–125.

Ryan, Kenneth, J; George, CR. Sherris Medical Microbiology: *An Introduction to Infectious Disease*. 4th ed. New York: McGraw-Hill, 2004: 727-730.

Sack, DA; Sack, RB; Nair, GB; Siddique, AK. Cholera. *Lancet.* 2004 363, 223–233

Sansonetti, PJ; Ryter, A; Clerc, P; Maruelli, AT; Mounier, J. Multiplication of Shigella flexneri within HeLa cells: lysis of the phagocytic vacuole and plasmid-mediated contact hemolysis. *Infect. Immun.* 1986 51, 461-469.

Sansonetti, PJ; Tran, VN; Egile, C. Rupture of the intestinal epithelial barrier and mucosal invasion by *Shigella flexneri*. *Clin. Infect. Dis.* 1999 28, 466–475.

Sarker, MR; Carman, RJ; McClane, BA. Inactivation of the gene (cpe) encoding Clostridium perfringens enterotoxin eliminates the ability of two cpe-positive C. perfringens type A human gastrointestinal disease isolates to affect rabbit ileal loops. *Mol. Microbiol.* 1999 33, 946– 958.

Savioli, L; Smith, H; Thompson, A. Giardia and Cryptosporidium join the 1 'Neglected Diseases Initiative'. *Trends Parasitol.* 2006 22, 203-208.

Schesser, K; Spiik, AK; Dukuzumuremyi, JM; Neurath, MF; Pettersson, S; Wolf-Watz, H. The *yopJ* locus is required for *Yersinia*-mediated inhibition of NF-kB activation and cytokine expression: YopJ contains a eukaryotic SH2-like domain that is essential for its repressive activity. *Mol. Microbiol.* 1998 28, 1067–1079

Sheikh, J; Czeczulin, JR; Harrington, S; Hicks, S; Henderson, IR; Le Bouguénec, C; Gounon, P; Phillips, A; Nataro, JP. A novel dispersin protein in enteroaggregative *Escherichia coli*. *J. Clin. Invest.* 2002 110, 1329-1337

Shogomori, H; Futerman, AH. Cholera toxin is found in detergent insoluble rafts/domains at the cell surface of hippocampal neurons but is internalized via a raft-independent mechanism. *J. Biol. Chem.* 2001 276, 9182–9188

Simon, D; David, J; Brandt, LJ. Studies on the pathogenesis of cryptosporidia-incuced diarrhea in HIV-infected individuals. *Am. J. Gastroenterol.* 1994 89, 2277-2278

Skelkvåle, R; Uemura, T. Experimental diarrhea in human volunteers following oral administration of Clostridium perfringens enterotoxin. *J. Appl. Bacteriol.* 1977 43, 281– 286.

Smith, HV; Corcoran, GD. New drugs and treatment for cryptosporidiosis. *Curr. Opin. Infect. Dis.* 2004 17, 557–564.

Sparks, SG; Carman, RJ; Sarker, MR; McClane, BA. Genotyping of enterotoxigenic *Clostridium perfringens* fecal isolates associated with antibioticassociated diarrhea and food poisoning in North America. *J. Clin. Microbiol.* 2001 39, 883-888.

Stanley Jr, SL. Amoebiasis. *Lancet.* 2003 361, 1025–1034

Stark, D; Beebe, N; Marriott, D; Ellis J; Harkness, J. Prospective study of the prevalence, genotyping, and clinical relevance of *Dientamoeba fragilis* infections in an Australian population. *J. Clin. Microbiol.* 2005 43, 2718-2723.

Steinthorsdottir, V; Halldorsson, H; Andresson, OS. Clostridium perfringens b-toxin forms multimeric transmembrane pores in human endothelial cells. *Microb. Pathog.* 2000 28, 45– 50.

Su, C; Brandt, LJ. *Escherichia coli* O157:H7 infection in humans. *Ann. Intern. Med.* 1995 123, 698-714

Suresh, K; Venilla, GD; Tan, TC; Rohela, M. In vivo encystation of Blastocystis hominis. *Parasitol. Res.* 2009 104, 1373-1380.

Thapar, N; Sanderson, IR. Diarrhoea in children: an interface between developing and developed countries. *Lancet.* 2004 363, 641-533

Thielman, NM; Guerrant, RL. Clinical practice. Acute infectious diarrhea. *N. Engl. J. Med.* 2004 350, 38-47

Tormo, R; Polanco, I; Salazar-Lindo, E; Goulet, O. Acute infectious diarrhoea in children: new insights in antisecretory treatment with racecadotril. *Acta Pædiatrica.* 2008 97, 1008–1015.

Uchiya, K. A *Salmonella* virulence protein that inhibits cellular trafficking. *EMBO J.* 1999 18, 3924–3933

van Hal, SJ; Stark, DJ; Fotedar, R; Marriott, D; Ellis, JT; Harkness, JL. Amoebiasis: current status in Australia. *MJA.* 2007 186, 412–416

Van Nhieu, GT; Caron E; Hall, A; Sansonetti, PJ. IpaC induces actin polymerization and Vesy, CJ; Peterson, WL. Review article: the management of Giardiasis. *Aliment. Pharmacol. Ther.* 1999 13, 843-850.

Vial, PA; Robins-Browne, R; Lior, H; Prado, V; Kaper, JB; Nataro, JP; Maneval, D; Elsayed, A; Levine, MM. Characterization of enteroadherentaggregative *coli*, a putative agent of diarrheal disease. *J. Infect. Dis.* 1988 158, 70-79

Wang, HH; Shieh, MJ; Liao, KF. A blind, randomized comparison of racecadotril and loperamide for stopping acute diarrhea in adults. *World J. Gastroenterol.* 2005 11, 1540-1543

Warny M and Kelly CP (2003) Pathogenicity of *Clostridium difficile* toxins. In *Microbial Pathogenesis and the Intestinal Epithelial Cell,* 503 (Ed. Hecht G) Washington, DC: ASM Press

Warny, M; Pepin, J; Fang, A; Killgore, G; Thompson, A; Brazier, J; Frost, E; McDonald, LC. Toxin production by an emerging strain of Clostridium difficile associated with outbreaks of severe disease in North America and Europe. *Lancet.* 2005 366, 1079-1084

Wilkins, TD; Tucker, KD. *C. difficile* toxin A uses gal-α1–3galβ1–4GlcNAC as a functional receptor. *Microecol. Ther.* 1989 19, 225–231

Winn Jr., Washington, Allen, S; Janda, W; Koneman, E; Procop, G; Schreckenberger, P; Woods, G. Koneman's Color Atlas and Textbook of Diagnostic Microbiology. 6th ed. Philadelphia: Lippincott Williams & Wilkins, 2006, 1267-1270.

Wolf, MK. Occurrence, distribution, and associations of O and H serogroups, colonization factor antigens, and toxins of enterotoxigenic *Escherichia coli*. *Clin. Microbiol. Rev.* 1997 10, 569-584

World Health Organization. WHO/Pan American Health Organization/UNESCO report of a consultation of experts on amoebiasis. *Wkly Epidemiol. Rec. WHO.* 1997 72, 97-99.

Zeile, WL; Purich, DL; Southwick, FS. Recognition of two classes of oligoproline sequences in profiling-mediated acceleration of actin-based Shigella motility. *J. Cell Biol.* 1996 133, 49-59.

Zimmer, V; Schilling, MK; Buecker, A; Lammer, F; Raedle, J. Chronic diarrhea responding to proton pump inhibitors: a clinical sign of Zollinger-Ellison syndrome. *Am. J. Med.* 2009 122, e9-e10.

Index

A

access, 38
acid, 8, 19, 28, 56
adaptability, 59
adenitis, 40
adenosine, 7, 14
adhesion, 18, 44
ADP, 13, 18, 20
age, 31, 39, 40, 42, 44
AIDS, 29, 30, 62
alcohol, 55
alters, 24
amebiasis, 46, 70
amino acids, 6, 7
angiotensin II, 15
anorexia, 25, 28, 29, 45
antacids, x, 4, 9
antibiotic, x, 21, 23, 35, 41, 44, 58, 59, 61, 62
antigen, 43
antimicrobial therapy, 19, 23, 24
anus, 10
apoptosis, 37, 39, 40, 62, 66
appendicitis, 40
arrest, 40
arthritis, 37, 43
asymptomatic, 29, 36, 44, 45, 46
ATP, 36

atrophy, 12
attachment, 20, 32, 33, 40

B

bacteremia, 19, 41
bacteria, x, 2, 8, 9, 11, 12, 13, 18, 32, 33, 34, 36, 37, 38, 40, 41, 42, 43, 48, 49, 50, 59, 63, 64
bacterial infection, 59
bacterium, 11, 19, 21, 22, 32, 33, 36, 40
beef, 42
behavior, 4
beverages, 48, 55
bile, ix, 8, 57
bile acids, 8, 57
binding, 18, 34, 56, 66
biopsy, xi, 53
birds, 42
bismuth, 20, 49, 57
bleeding, 45
blocks, 43
blood, ix, x, 3, 6, 8, 9, 17, 25, 27, 32, 34, 35, 37, 39, 45, 53
blood pressure, 53
blood stream, ix, 3
blood supply, x
bloodstream, 41
bowel, ix, 1, 5, 8, 18, 23, 30, 31, 35, 37, 46, 47, 49, 55, 56, 59, 69

C

burning, 28, 37

cadmium, 15
caffeine, x, 9
calcitonin, 8
calcium, 13, 26, 33
campylobacter, 41
campylobacter enteritis, 41
cancer, x
capillary, 6
carbohydrate, 3, 5, 20
carbohydrates, ix, 3, 5, 65
carcinoid syndrome, 8, 57, 68
carcinoma, 8
carrier, 44
castor oil, ix
cattle, 51
cell, x, 6, 7, 9, 12, 13, 20, 33, 34, 36, 37, 38, 39, 40, 42, 43, 62, 64, 67, 71
cell cycle, 40
cell death, 34, 37, 62
cell membranes, 36
cell surface, 71
cellulose, 70
cestodes, 14
channels, 7, 13
cheese, 4
children, 1, 14, 25, 26, 29, 36, 38, 39, 40, 42, 44, 45, 59, 61, 62, 63, 69, 72
cholera, ix, 6, 8, 12, 13, 17, 18, 19, 20, 26, 29, 69
chronic illness, 49
chyme, 7
circulation, 4, 12, 45
cirrhosis, 19, 66
classes, 73
classification, 53
cleaning, 22
clinical symptoms, 5
coffee, 48
colitis, 33, 38, 40, 45, 46, 66
colon, 2, 5, 8, 9, 10, 31, 42, 44
colonization, 18, 20, 64, 66, 73
colostrum, 30
community, 68
competition, 34
complications, 9, 37, 54
components, 22, 54
composition, 9, 55
compounds, 43
concentration, 5, 31
conductance, 57
confusion, 53
constipation, 28, 56
consumption, 19, 38, 39, 40
contamination, 23, 27, 39, 49
control, 67
cooking, 23, 42
cooling, 23
copper, 15
coupling, 6
cryptosporidium, 30
CTA, 18
culture, 33, 70
cyclosporiasis, 30, 63, 70
cystic fibrosis, 13, 71
cytokines, 35, 37, 38
cytoplasm, 36, 38
cytoskeleton, 36, 42
cytotoxicity, 37

D

death, 44
deaths, 8, 17, 19, 25, 36, 44
deficiencies, 5
degradation, 13, 21
dehydration, x, 19, 26, 29, 41, 50, 54, 62
delayed gastric emptying, 25
depolymerization, 36
destruction, x, 9, 12, 17, 31, 34, 37
developed countries, 1, 59, 72
developed nations, 27
developing countries, 14, 27, 30, 35, 59
diet, 30, 37
diffusion, 6
digestion, ix, 4, 10
digestive enzymes, 5, 10

direct action, 25
discomfort, 31
diseases, 21, 22, 60
disinfection, 22
disorder, 5
disseminate, 38
distress, 20, 69
distribution, 73
DNA damage, 40
dosage, 28
drinking water, 49
drug therapy, 54
drug use, 15
drugs, x, 9, 15, 31, 55, 56, 57, 58, 59, 72
duodenum, 18, 21, 22, 27
duration, x, 24, 28, 55, 56

E

earth, 29
eating, 21, 24, 28, 42
ecology, 70
egg, 28, 51
elaboration, 20
elderly, 1, 15, 25, 43, 58, 70
electrolyte, 6, 8, 9, 15, 18, 34, 38, 41, 54, 69
encoding, 71
endocarditis, 41
endorphins, 56
endothelial cells, 72
energy, 5
enkephalins, 57
enteritis, 21, 41, 64, 68
environment, 25
environmental contamination, 25
enzymes, 11, 25
epidemic, 24, 35
epidemiology, 61
epithelia, 64
epithelial cells, 7, 12, 13, 26, 29, 30, 32, 34, 36, 38, 39, 44, 57, 62, 63, 66
epithelium, 10, 12, 19, 27, 32, 33, 40, 41, 42
erythema nodosum, 40
erythrocytes, 70
ethanol, 5

etiology, 11, 53, 68
eukaryotic cell, 63, 66
evacuation, 10
excretion, 38, 44
exposure, 1, 35, 41, 68
extracellular matrix, 45

F

failure, 18, 43, 49
family, 64
fat, ix, 8
fatigue, 28, 30
fatty acids, ix, 5, 8, 68
feces, 25, 27, 29, 39, 41, 42, 44
fermentation, 13
fever, 12, 17, 19, 23, 25, 26, 27, 29, 30, 32, 33, 34, 35, 37, 38, 39, 40, 41, 43, 46, 47, 51, 56
fibrosis, 57
filament, 36
fish, 19, 49
flatulence, 37
flatworms, 14
flora, 21
fluid, x, 6, 8, 9, 11, 13, 15, 18, 20, 26, 29, 30, 34, 35, 38, 47, 51, 54, 63, 68, 69
follicles, 38
food, ix, 18, 19, 20, 21, 22, 23, 24, 27, 29, 30, 32, 36, 38, 41, 42, 44, 48, 49, 50, 55, 57, 61, 63, 64, 65, 66, 72
food poisoning, 21, 22, 23, 41, 50, 61, 64, 65, 66, 72
formula, 54
fruits, ix, 3, 49
fusion, 43

G

gastrin, 8
gastrinoma, ix
gastritis, 25
gastroenteritis, 10, 24, 25, 39, 40, 41, 44, 47, 69

gastrointestinal tract, 23
gene, 34, 36, 61, 62, 68, 71
gene expression, 34
generation, 7
genes, 45
genetics, 71
glucagon, 8
glucose, 5, 6, 7, 8, 13, 19, 26, 34, 54, 62
gout, 15
granules, 44
groups, 14
growth, 22, 34
gut, ix, 3, 10, 21, 24, 30, 31, 42, 58, 61, 66

H

habitat, 17
half-life, 57
halitosis, 28
hands, 25, 42
headache, 30, 41
health, 34, 36, 54
health care, 34
heat, 7, 20, 21, 23, 33, 50, 68
hemagglutinins, 18
heme, 53
hemolytic uremic syndrome, 37
HIV, 26, 62, 72
HIV-1, 26, 62
homosexuality, 59
hospitalization, 23, 26, 59
hospitals, 24, 26
host, 14, 29, 33, 36, 38, 39, 40, 42, 43, 45, 62, 63, 64
hotels, 49
hygiene, 27, 36, 48
hyperthyroidism, x, 9
hypotension, 12, 35

I

ileum, 10, 31
immune system, 12, 25, 43
immunity, 49

immunocompromised, 1, 20, 29, 30, 41
implementation, 67
incidence, 8, 36
incubation period, 25
induction, 13, 21
infants, 1, 20, 25, 68
infection, 19, 20, 24, 25, 27, 28, 29, 31, 33, 35, 36, 37, 40, 44, 46, 56, 61, 62, 65, 68, 69, 72
inflammation, 9, 17, 22, 31, 33, 34, 37, 38, 40, 42, 44, 45, 70
inflammatory cells, 9, 33
inflammatory mediators, 45
ingestion, 15, 18, 20, 21, 22, 23, 27, 29, 30, 32, 36, 42, 43, 44, 50
inhibition, 14, 29, 70, 71
inhibitor, 57
institutions, 35
interaction, 20, 62
interface, 72
interleukin-8, 66
intervention, 28
intestinal flora, 22
intestinal tract, 21, 42, 63, 68, 70
intestinal villi, 25
intestine, ix, x, 3, 4, 6, 7, 9, 10, 13, 29, 34, 54
intravenous antibiotics, 20
intravenous fluids, 26
invertebrates, 18
iodine, 48
ion transport, 64
ions, x, 4, 6, 62
iron, 15
ischemia, 39

J

jejunum, 18, 29, 71

K

killing, 58

L

lactase, 5, 55
lactase deficiency, 5, 55
lactic acid, 5
lactose, ix, 3, 5, 30, 55, 66
lactose intolerance, 5, 66
lakes, 27
large intestine, x, 13, 15, 33
laxatives, ix, x, 4, 9, 15
lesions, 1, 9, 23, 32, 33, 46
leukocytosis, 35
life cycle, 29
ligand, 20, 67
line, 28
liver, 22, 45, 46
liver abscess, 46
liver damage, 22
livestock, 27
localization, 65
locus, 62, 71
loss of appetite, 30, 43
lumen, ix, 3, 4, 5, 6, 7, 8, 9, 14, 18, 37, 42, 46
lymph, 39
lymph node, 39
lymphoid, 38
lymphoma, x, 9
lysis, 64, 71

M

macromolecules, 7
macrophages, 37, 39, 43
magnesium, x, 4, 9, 64
maintenance, 8
majority, 27
malabsorption, ix, 5, 25, 27, 29, 67
malaise, 22, 28, 39, 41, 47
malaria, 44
males, 1
malnutrition, 33
maltose, 7
management, 49, 54, 73
mannitol, 3, 4
matrix, 45, 68
measures, 36
meat, 23, 32, 39, 49
membranes, 62
men, 59
meningismus, 37
meningitis, 41
menstruation, 9
metabolic acidosis, 54
metabolism, 12, 66
mice, 62
microinjection, 39
microorganism, 35
milk, 5, 23, 32, 39, 42, 49, 50, 51
minority, 23
misconceptions, 66
molecules, 4, 7, 14, 39
morbidity, 1, 35
morphine, 56
morphology, 8, 10, 30
mortality, 1, 8, 22, 35, 46
mortality rate, 22, 46
motor activity, 10
movement, 9, 13, 49, 65
mucoid, 32, 45
mucosa, ix, x, 1, 6, 13, 17, 18, 30, 32, 33, 34, 35, 36, 40, 41, 45
mucous membrane, 53
mucous membranes, 53
mucus, 19, 29, 33, 35, 39, 45
multiplication, 21, 43
myalgia, 25
myosin, 63

N

NaCl, 7
nausea, 12, 15, 19, 21, 22, 23, 25, 28, 29, 30, 37, 41, 43, 47, 50, 57
nervous system, 26
neurons, 18, 72
neutrophils, 37, 38, 41
nontropical sprue, ix
normal distribution, 43

nuclei, 45
nutrients, 5, 7, 9, 34

O

observations, 44
obstruction, 8
ofloxacin, 49
opiates, 56, 57
orange juice, 54
organism, xi, 1, 11, 17, 20, 22, 23, 35, 39, 46, 47, 50, 51
osmolality, 4
oysters, 19

P

pain, 21, 23, 25, 31, 33, 40, 41, 45, 50, 57
pancreatic insufficiency, ix, 5
pancreatitis, 67, 70
parasite, 11, 29, 31, 44, 45, 70
parasitic infection, 9, 14
particles, 24, 25
passive, 71
pasta, 22
pathogenesis, 31, 43, 70, 71, 72
pathogens, 1, 12, 24, 32, 47, 53, 58, 59, 63, 64, 68
pathology, 34
pathophysiology, 64
peptides, 7, 18, 44
perforation, 37, 46
peristalsis, 56
peri-urban, 68
permeability, 8, 45
permission, iv
permit, 34
person-to-person contact, 24
phagocyte, 43
phagocytosis, 63
pharmacological research, 59
pharmacotherapy, 64
plasma, 19, 23, 32
plasma membrane, 19, 23, 32

plasmid, 38, 62, 71
polymerization, 38, 63, 73
pools, 32
poor, 27
population, 1, 27, 72
poultry, 42, 51
poverty, 59
pressure, 10, 24
prisons, 24
probiotic, 30, 35
production, 5, 11, 14, 33, 36, 38, 45, 68, 70, 73
properties, 24, 57, 64
prophylactic, 48
prostaglandins, x, 8, 9, 29
protein synthesis, 34, 37
proteins, x, 9, 14, 36, 39, 42, 43, 45, 67
proteolytic enzyme, 21
proton pump inhibitors, 15, 74
pseudomembranous colitis, 34, 35
pseudopodia, 37
public health, 67
pulse, 53
pumps, 7
purification, 48
pus, x, 8, 9, 17, 27, 32, 37, 45

R

rain, 27
range, 40
rash, 40
reason, 25
receptors, 37, 40, 56, 57, 69
recommendations, iv
recovery, 25, 50, 51
rectum, 63
recurrence, 35
refugee camps, 35
region, 2, 69
rehydration, 19, 49, 54, 55, 56, 59
reintroduction, 54
relapses, 41
relevance, 72
residues, 34

resistance, 45, 58
respiratory, 37
returns, 43
rice, 18, 22, 50
risk, 25, 61
risk factors, 61
room temperature, 23
rotavirus, 1, 12, 25, 26, 69
roundworms, 14

S

salicylates, 20
salmonella, 44
salt, 19, 50, 54, 55
salts, ix, 4
school, 35
seafood, 19
search, 59
secrete, 18, 20, 33, 37, 45
secretion, ix, 6, 7, 8, 11, 13, 15, 20, 26, 29, 33, 34, 37, 39, 43, 47, 56, 57, 63, 69
selective serotonin reuptake inhibitor, 15
sensitivity, 20, 57
sepsis, 41, 44
serotonin, x, 8, 9, 18, 57
serum, 9
severity, 36, 41, 45, 49, 53, 69
sewage, 42
sex, 44
shellfish, 19, 49
shock, 18, 35
side effects, 56, 60
sigmoidoscopy, xi, 53
signs, 39, 53
skin, 19, 53
small intestine, 5, 6, 10, 12, 19, 21, 22, 23, 26, 27, 29, 30, 33, 42, 47, 64
sodium, ix, 4, 6, 18, 19, 20, 26, 29, 62, 64
soil, 21, 27
space, 6, 34
species, 11, 14, 36, 38, 41
spectrum, 34
sphincter, 10, 67, 70
spore, 21, 22

starch, 22, 54
steatorrhea, 27
stomach, 7, 19, 22, 29, 37
stool culture, 53
storage, 19
strain, 36, 41, 73
strategies, 63, 67
submucosa, 39, 40
substrates, 4
sugar, 4, 54
sulfonamides, 42
surface area, 13
survival, 43, 44
susceptibility, 62
symptom, ix
symptomatic treatment, xi
symptoms, 1, 12, 14, 19, 21, 23, 24, 27, 31, 37, 40, 41, 43, 45, 46, 50
syndrome, 8, 22, 23, 25, 27, 33, 41, 50, 56

T

targets, 39
teeth, 48
teicoplanin, 58
temperature, 53
therapeutic agents, 46
therapeutic approaches, 60, 68
therapy, x, 18, 20, 22, 24, 35, 38, 41, 44, 48, 50, 54, 56, 59
threat, 42
thrombocytopenic purpura, 33
thrombophlebitis, 41
thyroid, 8
tincture, 20, 48
tissue, 33, 46, 70
TNF, 70
toxic megacolon, 20, 35, 56
toxic shock syndrome, 24
toxin, 6, 13, 18, 20, 21, 22, 23, 24, 26, 32, 33, 35, 37, 38, 40, 50, 63, 64, 65, 66, 67, 71, 72, 73
transcription, 34, 38
transmission, 24, 26, 27, 31, 44, 46, 59, 63
transport, 19, 26, 56, 65

triggers, 45
trypsin, 21
tuberculosis, x, 9
tumor, 35
tumor necrosis factor, 35
tumors, ix
tumours, 68
turgor, 53

U

ulcerative colitis, x, 9, 67
UNESCO, 73
urinary tract, 46
urine, 38

V

vaccine, 38, 49, 67
vacuole, 36, 38, 71
vagus, x, 9, 22
vagus nerve, x, 9
vancomycin, 35, 70
vasoactive intestinal peptide, 8, 10

vector, 34, 36
vegetables, 23, 42, 49, 50
vesicle, 43
victims, 23
villus, 6
viral infection, 29
viruses, x, 8, 11, 13, 24, 25, 26, 48
vomiting, 12, 15, 17, 19, 22, 23, 24, 25, 26, 27, 29, 30, 37, 39, 41, 43, 50, 51

W

water absorption, 19, 29
water quality, 49
water supplies, 27
weight loss, 28, 29, 30, 45
wild animals, 27
wind, 27
winter, 25

Z

zinc, 15